INTERPERSONAL PERCEPTION
A Social Relations Analysis

DISTINGUISHED CONTRIBUTIONS IN PSYCHOLOGY
A Guilford Series

Edited by
Kurt W. Fischer   E. Tory Higgins   Lawrence A. Pervin
Harvard University   *Columbia University*   *Rutgers University*

INTERPERSONAL PERCEPTION
A Social Relations Analysis
David A. Kenny

INTERPERSONAL PERCEPTION
A Social Relations Analysis

DAVID A. KENNY

Foreword by Harry T. Reis

THE GUILFORD PRESS
New York / London

*I dedicate this book to my
students and my graduate advisor,
Donald T. Campbell.
I owe everything to them.*

©1994 The Guilford Press
A Division of Guilford Publications, Inc.
72 Spring Street, New York, NY 10012

Printed in the United States of America

This book is printed on acid-free paper.

Last digit is print number: 9 8 7 6 5 4 3 2 1

Library of Congress Cataloging-in-Publication Data

Kenny, David A., 1946–
    Interpersonal perception : a social relations analysis /
David A. Kenny.
        p.   cm.
    Includes bibliographical references and index.
    ISBN 0-89862-114-3
    1. Social perception.   I. Title.
HM132.K454   1994
    302'.12—dc20   94-8552
                                                          CIP

SERIES EDITORS' NOTE

We believe that psychology is entering an exciting period. Increasingly, scholars in social, personality, developmental, cognitive, and other areas of psychology are moving away from investigating limited phenomena and issues constrained by disciplinary boundaries and toward the examination of basic psychological principles. This renewed interest in basic principles at multiple levels of analysis can serve to reunite the field of psychology. In addition, psychologists of all disciplines, both researchers and practitioners, can directly benefit from an understanding of the psychological principles being explored by their colleagues in other areas. It is the goal of the new Guilford series, "Distinguished Contributions in Psychology," to identify scholars whose unique perspective on a basic psychological principle makes their ideas essential reading to a broad range of other scholars in psychology and related fields.

This book by David Kenny represents an auspicious beginning to our new series. It presents an original and coherent statement on the nature of interpersonal perception in social interaction. The message is clear and powerful. The perspective is unique and insightful. The contribution is fundamental and potentially of historical significance. We are very pleased to have David Kenny's *Interpersonal Perception* launch what promises to be an exciting enterprise.

Kurt W. Fischer
E. Tory Higgins
Lawrence A. Pervin

FOREWORD

I n the early days of contemporary social psychology, person perception was one of the emerging discipline's core phenomena. Those
pioneering researchers knew that there was something special about
ways in which we come to know about other persons, and that this
"something special" distinguished our perception of people from our
perception of objects. This may be one of those instances in which,
to amend the biologist Ernst Haeckel's time-honored axiom, episte-
mology recapitulates ontogeny. One of the first cognitive challenges
that newborn babies master is the ability to discriminate people from
other objects in the environment. Later on, of course, this task becomes more complex. People can be characterized on more dimensions
than Heinz has varieties and Baskin-Robbins has flavors. The task of
the social perceiver is to create sensible, stable, personally useful, and
(possibly) accurate representations of others, especially of those who
occupy prominent roles in our lives. In other words, our beliefs about
others, be they right or wrong, have important implications for social
interaction.

Interpersonal perception, as David Kenny refers to it, grew out
of social psychology's durable tradition of person perception research.
To appreciate the novelty and insightfulness of his approach, the reader
needs to understand its roots. Person perception research evolved out
of psychology's fascination with an intrinsically compelling question:
Can a person accurately perceive another person's traits, abilities, and
emotions? Not surprisingly, this question did not yield simple answers.
Perhaps as a result, researchers like Solomon Asch and Fritz Heider
took a different and less direct tack, one that predominates to this day.
They investigated the processes by which people form impressions of
others, presumably anticipating that by identifying these processes, the
sources of accuracy and inaccuracy ultimately would be illuminated.

A focus on process, together with the experimentalist's passion
for control over relevant variables, underlies the extensive existing
literature. Although much of this research uses vignettes — which, as

Kenny aptly notes, bypass most of the richness and complexity inherent in everyday person perception — we should not overlook the tangible benefits that this approach has generated during the past half century of scholarly activity. Every introductory social psychology textbook summarizes an elaborate and bountiful store of empirical findings and theoretical models characterizing the manner in which people form impressions of others, as well as the many diverse factors that influence these judgments. Nevertheless, it is time for a model that is truly interpersonal, interactive, and reflective. This book describes such a model.

Other researchers persevered on questions of accuracy and inaccuracy, notably Lee Cronbach, who, in a seminal 1955 paper, showed that accuracy was not a simple matter of computing a difference score between a subject's standing on some trait (say, intelligence) and a judge's rating of that subject on that trait. Cronbach's paper showed that thoughtful analysis, mixed with a little bit of mathematics, goes a long way (thereby verifying the homilies many of us endured in high-school algebra). That is, he demonstrated that accuracy judgments of this sort were actually an imprecise conglomeration of four independent components, which he labeled *elevation, differential elevation, stereotype accuracy,* and *differential accuracy.* (Kenny explains these four components far better than I can, and I refer eager readers to Chapter 7.) If not identified and assessed, these four components combine in unknown and potentially countervailing ways, yielding scores with obscure meaning and studies with ambiguous findings.

Cronbach's paper marked a watershed in the history of person perception research — indeed, it was recently honored as one of "top 10" most cited papers in 40 years of one of psychology's most prestigious journals, *Psychological Bulletin.* Unfortunately, Cronbach's critique, far from pointing researchers in the right direction, appears to have scared them off. The reasons for this departure are not clear, but complexity is probably one of them. (A historical irony is that, three years later, Cronbach disavowed some of the new indices that he proposed. The substance of his critique nevertheless remains valid.) To our enduring good fortune, not everyone was daunted by Cronbach's analysis; some, including David Kenny, took it as a clarion call to find new and better ways of studying such fundamental questions. This exciting new book is the result of Kenny's two-decade-long pursuit of these phenomena. If my hunch is correct, it will provide the beacon that entices researchers to the mainland of interpersonal perception research.

Readers must ask two questions when evaluating the significance of any new contribution to the literature. The first is, why does the subject of this book, interpersonal perception, matter? Second, what is novel and important about this particular approach to interpersonal perception? Answering the first question is easy. Interpersonal perception is indisputedly a central issue in social psychology. This is not merely a coincidence of history and tradition; it directly reflects the impact of interpersonal perception on virtually the entire panoply of phenomena in which social psychologists are interested. Consider, for example, the first two sections of the *Journal of Personality and Social Psychology,* the field's preeminent outlet for empirical research. One is entitled "attitudes and social cognition," the other is "interpersonal relations and group processes." The substance of interpersonal perception provides a conceptual bridge between these two outposts of our discipline.

We might also gauge the centrality of interpersonal perception to social psychology by imagining the list of topics and processes that cannot be fully understood without recourse to basic principles of interpersonal perception. One thinks readily of stereotypes, first impressions, interpersonal attraction, behavioral confirmation, attributions, social identity, self-perception and reflected appraisal, intimacy and responsiveness, social comparison, nonverbal communication, meta-communication, conformity and social influence, and leadership, to name some obvious examples. If interpersonal perception was not already a major heading in the social psychological catalog, we would surely have to go out and invent it!

Readers would better appreciate my comments on the second above question as an epilogue to this volume, not a foreword. Nevertheless, because it is often easier to begin a journey with a few visible milestones, I offer a few general thoughts here. Kenny's Social Relations Model (SRM) approach is the only research strategy available to person perception researchers that is explicitly designed to capitalize on two fundamental facts of social life: that interaction is always bidirectional, and that people reflect on their interactions. That is, while Person A is busy sizing up Person B, B is at the same moment assessing A. Furthermore, while thinking about the other, both persons are likely to be wondering what the other is thinking about them. (As Bette Midler once said, "That's enough talk about me. Let's talk about you. What do you think of me?") In the past, researchers usually had to ignore these all-important considerations, not because they were unaware of them (our scholarly foreparents were too smart for that!), but because they lacked an unimpeachable means for addressing such complexities. SRM provides such a tool, and the result is described in this book.

The architect Ludwig Mies van der Rohe is reputed to have said,

"God is in the details." Social relations analysis is not only about getting the details; it is about getting them right. This is evident in the
systematic and painstaking way in which Kenny poses, frames, and
then examines nine basic questions of interpersonal perception. Consider reciprocity, a phenomenon in which researchers from many disciplines have long been interested. Social relations analysis instructs
us that reciprocity is not one question, but two: "Do A and B see each
other similarly?" is distinct from "Does A think B sees A in the same
way A sees B?" Moreover, social relations analysis further informs us
that answering the first question is (alas) not a simple matter of asking A and B how they perceive each other, and correlating their
responses. That is because, as the reader will discover in Chapter 2,
each of these ratings incorporates three systematic sources of variance:
perceiver effects, target effects, and relationship effects. Failing to
separate these components provides data that are inherently confounded, and findings that are in all likelihood destined to be ambiguous.
That is why it is so important to regard interpersonal perception in
the degree of detail that Kenny proposes.

Or consider the accuracy question with which this field got its
start, more than a half century ago. Kenny's analysis indicates that
what we naively think of as a single construct, accuracy, is actually
a series of questions, each describing one particular kind of accuracy.
For example, there is generalized target accuracy, knowing how another
persons typically behaves. And there is also dyadic target accuracy,
knowing how another person is likely to behave with oneself. Existing paradigms have not only kept us from discriminating these questions empirically, incidentally, but have, more consequentially, kept
our theorizing in conceptual blinders. Our scholarship has for the most
part tended to merge these phenomena. Not that we should not have
known better, of course: In real life, we all know someone who is generally shy and aloof, but open and friendly with ourselves. Sorting out
these distinctions is what the social relations approach is all about.

A great strength of this book is that it systematically pulls together
existing studies that take a social relations approach to these nine basic
questions of interpersonal perception. By posing and beginning to answer these vital questions, Kenny's synthesis will surely benefit the field.
A potentially greater contribution is the method itself. The social relations model offers a rigorous and innovative method for studying
most, if not all, interpersonal phenomena. Researchers who study the
diverse phenomena of attraction, communication, interaction, and relationships have lacked paradigms for identifying and isolating the various components that contribute to a given observation. Consider a
single data point: Jack loves Jill. Is this because Jack generally loves

others? Is it because people generally love Jill? Or is it because there is something about Jack's feelings for Jill that transcends his usual lovingness and her typical lovability? A moment's reflection reveals that the conceptual implications of this distinction are more significant than mere methodological refinements would be. That is, substantive conclusions about this data point will vary markedly, depending on which interpretation is the right one.

Thus, one model that Kenny describes in this book should have widespread appeal across various substantive interests and disciplinary boundaries. The method can enhance the internal and ecological validity of interpersonal research, a considerable contribution in itself. Interpersonal researchers sometimes feel compelled to choose between drawing cautious, scientifically valid inferences on one hand, and studying natural, involving, and contextually embedded behavior on the other. Much as for the ancient Greek sailors who found themselves between Scylla the rock and Charibdis the whirlpool, either emphasis may heighten vulnerability to the other danger. This is of course not a very satisfactory state of affairs as we enter the second half century of research. Fortunately, methods are emerging that obviate the need for such choices, and social relations analysis is one of the best of them.

I am reluctant to taint this innovative and thoughtful work (in the eyes of some) by describing it as a new "research method." The methodological label sometimes carries the unfortunate connotation of a focus on technique and procedure, rather than concepts, theories and substance—that it is, in simpler language, "technical fussing." Such an inference would be short sighted, misleading, and just plain wrong. This "method" is based on a sophisticated understanding of how social behavior derives from an intricate synthesis of *reaction* and *inter*-action. It is a tool capable of unraveling complex phenomena and providing genuinely new insights into social perception and behavior. The method is about asking better questions of our data, and obtaining more precise knowledge from our investigations. Surely our mission as researchers demands no less.

As Asch pointed out nearly a half century ago, "this remarkable capacity we possess to understand something of the character of another person . . . is a precondition of social life" (1946, p. 258). Past research has taught us much about the manner in which people perceive one another, and the implications of interpersonal perception for a host of social psychological phenomena. The research summarized in this book provides a major stepping stone toward the next generation of studies. It also has potential applications that even Kenny himself may not have realized. In the *Terminator* movies, cyborgs come equipped with a complex sensing system that allows them to instantaneously assess various characteristics of the persons they encounter. I have a strong hunch that the central components of these systems are a 21st-century update of the model of interpersonal perception that David Kenny describes herein. This is just conjecture, however; what is certain is that readers will find intellectual challenge and excitement in the pages that follow.

Harry T. Reis
University of Rochester

ACKNOWLEDGMENTS

The idea for this book has its roots in my original interest in psychology. Getting to know others and ourselves is fascinating; it is something that we all do. To be able to study this as my livelihood was what initially attracted me to psychology. However, most of my early work had little to do with person perception. I had trouble determining how to study this topic with the tools that I was learning. So, during my graduate career, I concentrated on the study of methodology under the able tutelage of Donald T. Campbell. Ironically, most of what I learned from Campbell about interpersonal perception came after I left graduate school.

At Harvard in the mid- to late 1970s, work with Rebecca Warner, Jeffrey Berman, and Pierce Barker caused me to return to my original interests. But it was not until moving to the University of Connecticut in 1978 and collaborating with Lawrence La Voie that I really returned to this topic. La Voie and I devised the "Social Relations Model" (SRM), and developed many important uses of the model. SRM is the product of my work *and* La Voie's, not just my own. Subsequent work with other graduate students at Connecticut, especially Thomas Malloy, Linda Albright, and Deborah Kashy, greatly expanded the potential use of the SRM.

Critical in the development of the approach was a sabbatical year at the Center for Advanced Studies in the Behavioral Sciences at Stanford, and a year's leave of absence spent at Arizona State. These two years gave me the time to develop computer software. Also at Arizona State, feedback from Doug Kenrick, Steve West, Sandy Braver, and Nancy Eisenberg was especially helpful.

Besides institutional support, the work required financial assistance. I have been supported for most of the last 15 years by the National Science Foundation. Also, for a three-year period I received a grant from the National Institute of Mental Health. It permitted me to hire a postdoctoral assistant, Linda Acitelli, who has broadened my thinking about two-person relationships in numerous ways.

I have collaborated with many individuals in data collection. Among them are Peter Oliver, Nancy Bernstein, Caryl Horner, Ling-chuan Chu, Andrea Chapdelaine, Maurice Levesque, Patrick Sullivan, Suzanne Kieffer, and Kathyrn LaFontana. Even more numerous are those who have given me access to data that they have collected with great difficulty and effort. Among these are Donald T. Campbell, Jim Dabbs, Ray Reno, Bella DePaulo, Ross Buck, Bernadette Park, Julie Yingling, Mick Rothbart, Daniel Thomsen, Debby Moskowitz, Vicky McGillan, Barbara Montgomery, and Bibb Latané.

Numerous colleagues have also provided support and criticism. Very early on, an encouraging letter by Theodore Newcomb was very gratifying. I owe a great deal to Barbara Montgomery, who opened up to me the possibility of using rating data within SRM. Criticisms by Loring Ingraham and Tom Wright, though stinging at the time, did reorient me in appropriate ways. Numerous conversations with Charles Judd and Bernadette Park were critical in reshaping my thinking and pushing me in directions that I never would have had the courage to pursue alone. Also, through the years, Harold Kelley has been very supportive.

Nearly every day, I had the opportunity to share my ideas with Reuben Baron. Other colleagues at Connecticut, particularly Skip Lowe, Ross Buck, Greg Hixon, and Jim Green, have also served as valuable sounding boards. Very significantly, Jerry Smith and Ron Growney as department chairs and Amerigo Farina as associate chair made Connecticut the right place to do this work.

Clerical assistance has been essential throughout this entire effort, particularly from Alice Mellian during the mid-1970s, Robyn Ireland during the early 1980s, and my current secretary, Virginia Carrow. They have suffered though numerous drafts and dealt with complicated symbols. Garvin Boudle also provided important assistance in the preparation of the figures.

I am extremely grateful to the reviewers of this book. James Uleman, Harry Reis, Charles Bond, Maurice Levesque, Kathryn LaFontana, and Tom Malloy read the the entire book. Bill Swann, Skip Lowe, Bernadette Park, Mary Ellen Kenny, and Lynn Winquist read selected chapters. They were diligent in finding errors and urging me to clarify obscure passages. Also Kathryn LaFontana was especially helpful during the final stages of preparation of the manuscript.

My family has been supportive in this process. My children, none of whom was even born when I started this project, have read various parts of this book. My wife, Mary Ellen, has put up with the late hours, the conventions, and the time that I have been in her presence but lost in the pages of this book.

CONTENTS

The Notational System, 216
Behavior and Perception, 217
Postscript, 225

Chapter 1

INTRODUCTION

People all have beliefs about the other people that they know. A woman might believe that her parents are harsh, that her lover is kind, and that her friend is intelligent. These beliefs guide people in various ways. They help people predict and explain the behavior of others. A man may believe that because his girlfriend is intelligent, she can do complicated crossword puzzles. Beliefs about others are also useful when one person has to describe another person to a third party. However, their primary utility lies in helping people guide their interactions with others. Beliefs about others tell people whom they should avoid, with whom they should leave their car when they go on a long trip, whom they should date, and whom they should ask for advice when they have a personal problem. So people's beliefs about others have important consequences in their everyday lives.

Within social psychology, the study of the beliefs that people have about others is called "person perception." Technically, many beliefs that a person has about another are not perceptions, but rather are inferences or the result of communication from others. For instance, people may infer that because someone is young, he or she is adventurous. Adventurousness is not perceived; rather, it is inferred. Also, if John tells Mary that Scott is intelligent, Mary's belief that Scott is intelligent is not a perception because it is not based on direct observation. Nonetheless, the tradition within social psychology is to refer to these beliefs as "person perceptions."

Person perception is fundamentally different from object perception in at least four ways. First, person perception is reciprocal. A person may perceive a chair as soft, brown, and maybe even friendly (in the sense of comfortable), but the chair does not perceive the person back. Object perception is one-sided: A person perceives the object, but the object does not perceive the person. Person perception is generally two-sided: People perceive each other. The two-sided nature of person perception means that people are simultaneously "checking each other out."

A second difference between person and object perception is as follows: When I encounter another person, not only is the other perceiving me; I also know that the other is doing so, and I wonder how he or she sees me. People spend a great deal of their time trying to read other people's minds. This is particularly salient during a job interview or a first date. Even when people are engaged in ordinary, everyday interactions, they often say to themselves, "I wonder if he took that the wrong way?" or "I must have looked really stupid." Very often, people also care strongly about whether other persons really like them. If people believe that other persons do not like them, they may adjust their behavior accordingly.

Another way in which person perception differs from object perception is that person perception is directly tied to self-perception, whereas in object perception, self-perception is much less important. In perceiving others, people may imagine others as similar to them—something not usually done in object perception. Moreover, how people think that others see them is probably directly tied to self-perception. So self-perception is closely linked to person perception, and it is not as closely linked to object perception.[1]

Finally, person perception differs from object perception because people change much more than physical objects do. Generally, the color, shape, and size of a physical object are very stable. But the behavior of people is quite variable and changeable. An individual's behavior changes when he or she is with different interaction partners. A child may be quiet and obedient when with a parent, but wild and aggressive when with peers. Characteristics of objects are generally permanent, whereas people are quite variable. Although it is true that people often do not seem to recognize the fact that others are quite variable (something called "correspondence bias" or the "fundamental error of attribution"), it is still essential that models of interpersonal perception allow for the possibility of change.

The Traditional Research Paradigm

Traditionally, person perception research in social psychology has treated people much as if they were physical objects. Social psychologists typically study person perception by presenting people with little stories, called "vignettes," about a hypothetical person and then asking them what they think about the person in the vignette. For instance, a subject in an experiment might receive the following vignette: "Zelda Brown is a librarian at the local high school. She likes to go dancing at night, and she favors many very conservative political positions." Often these vignettes are presented in a very skeletal form: "Zelda Brown: librarian, party animal, politically conservative."

Social psychologists use vignettes, as opposed to having research participants actually interact, for two reasons. First, with a vignette the exact information that a person receives from the interaction partner can be controlled. For instance, if researchers want to know the effect of physical appearance on person perception, they can present people with information about hair color and weight and see how that information affects judgments. In this way, the researchers know exactly what information people get when they "observe" the other. There is no need to worry about the people paying attention to other "irrelevant information" such as age, because age information is not given. Second, a researcher can present a person with many (e.g., 20) of these vignettes in an hour, whereas it would be impossible to have the person interact with that many people in an hour. So vignette research allows for greater control of stimulus information and is more efficient than research that permits the person to interact with the other. For these reasons, the use of vignettes has been the norm in person perception research.[2]

Although the field of social psychology has learned much from vignette research, this type of research fails to capture the important richness of everyday person perception. Person perception in vignette research is one-sided: The research participant perceives the target in the vignette, but the target does not perceive the perceiver. Also, the perceiver does not engage in mind reading. He or she does not wonder how the target in the vignette sees him or her. (Interestingly, participants in research do play mind games with the experimenter. They are very concerned about how the experimenter evaluates them.)

I use the term "interpersonal perception" to distinguish it from the usual person perception in vignette research. In interpersonal perception research, the perceiver and the target are allowed to interact with each other. Moreover, the two form impressions about each other. In addition to these impressions, self-perceptions and perceptions about how a person thinks others see him or her are often measured. Interpersonal perception research captures the richness of perceiving other people. More details are given about interpersonal perception research in this and the next chapter.

Compared with the traditional paradigm, interpersonal perception research does result in a loss of control of important variables. It cannot stand alone. It must be complemented by research that uses the traditional paradigm.

Types of Perceptions

Consider two people interacting: Zelda and Heidi are sitting in a doctor's waiting room, and they begin a conversation. There are three different types of perceptions: other-perception, meta-perception, and self-perception. First, they can perceive each other: Heidi may see Zelda as a relaxed, intelligent woman, whereas Zelda may see Heidi as boring and conventional. These are called "other-perceptions" or simply "perceptions." (The term "other-perception" is somewhat awkward, but a term is needed to distinguish ordinary perception of others from different types of perceptions. "Other-perception" should be read as "the perception of the other.") The two women may also engage in mind reading, and each may attempt to discern how she is seen by the other. For example, Zelda may wonder whether Heidi thinks that she is fat and old. These perceptions are called "reflected appraisals" or "meta-perceptions." There is a third type of perception: Zelda and Heidi engage in "self-perceptions." For instance, Heidi may see herself as witty and charming.

In interpersonal perception, there is a "perceiver" who rates a "target" on a given "trait." So if Heidi thinks that Zelda is lazy, Heidi is the perceiver, Zelda is the target, and the trait is laziness. As a second example, if Paul thinks that Ron is friendly, then Paul is the perceiver, Ron is the target, and the trait is friendliness. For self-perception, the perceiver and target are the same person. For meta-perception, matters are more complicated: If Zelda thinks that Heidi thinks that Zelda is intelligent, Zelda is the perceiver, Heidi is the target, and the trait is reflected intelligence. One might think that Heidi is the perceiver, but the person who has the perception is Zelda and not Heidi. Heidi is the target, in that the focus is her perception of Zelda. So for meta-perception, the perceiver and target in the other-perception are reversed. As a second example, if Paul thinks that Tom thinks that Paul is crazy, then Paul is the perceiver, Tom is the target, and reflected craziness is the trait.

The focus in this book is on the perception of traits such as friendliness, intelligence, and sociability. To what extent are traits important in people's perceptions of others? There are two sources of evidence that point to the importance of traits. First, if people are asked to describe people that they know, the bulk of their descriptions are traits. For instance, Fiske and Cox (1979) found that the dominant way in which people described others was with traits. So people spontaneously use traits in describing others. Second, when people observe the behavior of others but are not given a verbal trait label, there is strong evidence from memory data that they store the information about the others as a trait (Winter & Uleman, 1984). So it is reasonable to believe that traits are useful ways in which people understand each other.

It is helpful to develop a very simple notational system to capture the differences among other-perception, self-perception, and meta-perception. Let me call Zelda Z and call Heidi H. The symbol $Z(H)$ represents Zelda's perception of Heidi; in other words, the person outside the parentheses is the perceiver, and the person inside the parentheses is the target. As another example, $H(Z)$ represents Heidi's perception of Zelda. Reflected appraisal or meta-perception is given by $Z(H(Z))$, which represents Zelda's perception of Heidi's perception of Zelda. In self-perception, the perceiver and the target are the same persons, so the symbol of Heidi's perception of herself is $H(H)$. With this notation, it is possible to represent what a person thinks another thinks of a third person — $Z(H(C))$ — and how a person thinks another person views himself or herself — $Z(H(H))$. But this book concentrates on the meta-perception of what person Z thinks that another thinks about person Z, or $Z(H(Z))$.

A final symbol is needed that reflects the person's actual standing on the trait. Say there is an interest in how intelligent Zelda is. The symbol Z with no parentheses denotes Zelda's actual standing on the trait. To summarize, the basic symbols are as follows:

Other-perception: $Z(H)$ and $H(Z)$
Meta-perception: $Z(H(Z))$ and $H(Z(H))$
Self-perception: $Z(Z)$ and $H(H)$
Actual standing: Z and H

Basic Questions in Interpersonal Perception

Now that symbols have been developed for the different types of perceptions that people can have, the issue is how these perceptions are interrelated. The relationships among these perceptions give rise to the nine fundamental questions of interpersonal perception.

These nine fundamental questions are listed in Table 1.1. (Readers should refer to this table as necessary throughout the book.) I originally developed this list (Kenny, 1988), but it was based on the pioneering work of the social psychologists Tagiuri, Bruner, and Blake (1958); the psychoanalyst Laing (Laing, Phillipson, & Lee, 1966); the sociologist Scheff (1967); and the communication scientists McLeod and Chaffee (1973). The study of interpersonal perception is truly an interdisciplinary effort. Seven of the nine basic questions are my formulation (Kenny, 1988); two were added by Malloy and Albright (1990).

TABLE 1.1. Nine Basic Questions of Interpersonal Perception

Question	Statement	Symbol
Assimilation	Does Z see others as alike?	$Z(H) = Z(C)$
Consensus	Is H seen the same way by others?	$Z(H) = C(H)$
Uniqueness	Does Z see H idiosyncratically?	$Z(H) <> Z(C)$
		$Z(H) <> C(H)$
Reciprocity	Do Z and H see each other similarly?	$Z(H) = H(Z)$
Target accuracy	Is Z's view of H correct?	$Z(H) = H$
Assumed reciprocity	Does Z think others see her as she sees them?	$Z(H(Z)) = Z(H)$
Meta-accuracy	Does Z know how she is seen?	$Z(H(Z)) = H(Z)$
Assumed similarity	Does Z see others as she sees herself?	$Z(Z) = Z(H)$
Self–other agreement	Do others see Z as she sees herself?	$Z(Z) = H(Z)$

Note. The symbols, Z, H, and C stand for persons. The equal sign is meant to symbolize some correspondence and not exact agreement, and the symbol "< >" means "not equal." The table has been adapted from Kenny (1988). Copyright 1988 by Sage Publications, Ltd. Adapted by permission.

Although Table 1.1 provides a beneficial summary of the basic questions in person perception, it is quite dense. A complete explication of the questions requires reading the entire book.

Imagine three people, Zelda, Heidi, and Carol, who are denoted as *Z, H,* and *C,* respectively. Consider their perceptions of laziness. The first question presented in Table 1.1 is "assimilation." Does Zelda think that both Heidi and Carol are lazy? Assimilation means that a perceiver sees two targets as similar. The second question is "consensus": Do Zelda and Carol agree about how lazy Heidi is? Consensus concerns whether two perceivers agree when they judge a common target. The third question is "uniqueness": If Zelda's perception of Heidi show neither assimilation nor consensus effects, it can be said that Zelda's perception of Heidi is unique. Uniqueness concerns the extent to which a perceiver views a target idiosyncratically. The fourth question is "reciprocity": Do Heidi and Zelda see each other in the same way? So if Zelda thinks that Heidi is lazy, does Heidi think that Zelda is lazy? The first four questions—assimilation, consensus, uniqueness, and reciprocity—concern the degree of similarity or lack thereof between two other-perceptions.

The traditional accuracy question in person perception concerns the validity of other-perception. That is, if Zelda thinks that Heidi is lazy, is Heidi actually a lazy person? The validity of other-perception is called "target accuracy."

The next two questions, "assumed reciprocity" and "meta-accuracy," concern the degree of similarity between other-perception and meta-perception. Assumed reciprocity concerns the following question: If Zelda thinks that Heidi is lazy, does Zelda think that Heidi sees her as lazy? So do people think that others see them as they see others? The meta-accuracy question concerns the extent to which people are good mind readers: Does Zelda know that Heidi thinks that Zelda is a lazy person? Do people know what others think of them?

The last two questions, "assumed similarity" and "self–other agreement," concern the relationship between self-perception and other-perception. Assumed similarity concerns the relationship between how a person sees others and how the person sees himself or herself: Does Zelda think that people are similar to her? Self–other agreement refers to the correspondence between how others see a person and how that person sees himself or herself: If Heidi thinks that Zelda is lazy, does Zelda also see herself as lazy?

These are the nine fundamental questions in interpersonal perception. The purpose of this book is to present the best available evidence concerning these nine questions. These questions certainly do not exhaust the extent of possible questions in interpersonal perception. For instance, it can be asked to what degree meta-perceptions correspond to self-perceptions. But the line must be drawn somewhere, and so in this book the focus is on the nine questions; only occasionally does the book examine other questions when they provide information relevant to the nine basic questions.

It should also be realized that the questions are not independent. Sometimes the existence of one phenomenon precludes the existence of another. For instance, if there is perfect consensus, then there can be neither assimilation nor uniqueness. In other cases, the presence of certain phenomena implies others. For instance, if there are reciprocity and assumed reciprocity, there must be meta-accuracy. Finally, some phenomena require the existence of others. For instance, self–other agreement requires the existence of consensus.

The terms that are used in this book are somewhat arbitrary. For instance, assumed reciprocity has been called "congruence," and assumed similarity has been called "false-consensus bias." However, to avoid confusion, I exclusively use the terms in Table 1.1.

Research Evidence

Earlier, the typical research study in person perception—the vignette study—has been discussed. In this type of study, information about a fictitious person is presented to perceivers, who are asked to make judgments about the target. To study interpersonal perception, a different research paradigm must be used. First, people must serve as both perceivers and targets. Second, there must be an allowance for the possibility of meta-perception. Third, besides other-perception, self-perception must also be measured. Fourth, it should be taken into account that a person's behavior changes as a person interacts with different others. A paradigm called the "Social Relations Model" (SRM), which can accomplish these goals, is presented in Chapter 2.

Levels of Acquaintance

Typically, in studies of person perception, the target of perception is not a real person; it is a "paper person" defined by a list of traits or an actor in a videotape. Even if the target is a real person, the perceiver and target generally have no interaction history. However, in the studies to be described in this book, the level of acquaintance may range from none whatever (i.e., the perceiver and target are strangers) to lifelong friendship. It is useful to make the following distinctions in terms of describing the degree of acquaintance between perceiver and target.

First, there is zero acquaintance: The perceiver and target have never met, but the perceiver observes the target. For instance, a person is sitting in a restaurant and sees another person sitting across the room. It is easy to imagine what kind of person he or she is. For zero acquaintance, perception is often one-sided: Zelda views Heidi, but Heidi does not view Zelda. Although it is not interpersonal, zero acquaintance serves as an important baseline in the measurement of interpersonal perception.

Second, there is short-term acquaintance, in which people interact for a few minutes or hours. These interactions can be of two types: People may interact together in a group, or they may be separated into pairs and interact one-on-one, dyadically.

Third, there is long-term acquaintance, in which people know each other for a long time—perhaps years. This type of acquaintance can be broken into group and one-on-one interactions, but usually it is mixed. That is, people interact one-on-one at times and in larger groups at times. A prototypical study of this type is a study of the perceptions of sorority and fraternity members.

Trait Classification

As stated earlier, people commonly structure their knowledge about people around traits. Typically, most studies in person perception ask perceivers to rate the targets on scales. Rarely are perceivers asked to provide a free description of the target. Although free descriptions provide a rich source of data, it takes much longer to organize and analyze such data. Moreover, much (though not all) of the information from a free description can be much more economically obtained from trait rating scales.

In most studies of person perception, a good many traits are measured. For instance, in one important study (Park & Judd, 1989), 68 different traits were measured. Some way of collapsing results across traits is needed to make sense out of a mass of results. This book uses a classification system developed by Norman (1963), Goldberg (1990), Costa and McCrae (1985), and many others. This system has become known as the "Big Five." Although there is debate about the number of factors that are needed to describe personality (Zuckerman, Kuhlman, Joireman, Teta, & Kraft, 1993), the Big Five is the most common formulation.

Within the Big Five, both peer ratings and self-ratings of personality form five relatively independent factors:

Extroversion: How outgoing and animated is the person?
Agreeableness: How pleasant and positive is the person?
Conscientiousness: How conventional and hard-working is the person?
Emotional Stability: How relaxed and stable is the person?
Culture: How intelligent and sophisticated is the person?

Procedures for the classification of traits into the Big Five are presented elsewhere (Kenny, Albright, Malloy, & Kashy, in press).

Certainly the Big Five do not exhaust all the information about a person. But they do serve as a convenient way to categorize trait ratings. So a typical study that is considered in this book involves a group of people who meet, interact, and then rate one another on the Big Five factors.

In addition to questions related to the Big Five, perceivers are also often asked how much they like each target. Liking or affect is an important part of person perception, and its role in interpersonal perception is also considered.

Overview of the Book

A preview of each of the remaining nine chapters is presented here. Eight of the nine chapters concern theoretical issues, for which the relevant research evidence is presented.

Chapter 2: Methodology

Before a discussion of the nine questions is begun, it is necessary to present the general model that is used to answer the questions — the Social Relations Model (SRM). In this model, each perceiver rates multiple targets, and each target is rated by multiple perceivers. A key feature of the model is that it makes a distinction between two levels in person perception: the individual and the relationship. For instance, Zelda may think that Heidi is friendly because everyone sees Heidi that way (the person level), or because Zelda sees Heidi in a unique, idiosyncratic fashion (the relationship level). So Chapter 2 details issues concerning what data are collected, how they are interpreted, how they are analyzed, and what statistical summaries are to be presented.

Chapter 3: Assimilation

The colloquial way in which the assimilation question can be phrased is "Do they all look alike?" There is very strong evidence that people tend to see other people as more similar than they really are. A key issue concerns whether this tendency has a psychological meaning or whether it merely reflects how people use numbers when they rate others. Evidence is presented in Chapter 3 to support the position that people do assimilate and that assimilation reflects the assumptions made by perceivers about targets.

Assimilation reflects stereotypes that people have formed about other people. So if a person generally thinks that others are stupid (a stereotype), the person should rate people as low in intelligence. The stereotype develops from two different sources: significant others that the person has known in life, and the person's own self. Alternatively, assimilation effects can be viewed as reflections of more local stereotypes that perceivers have formed about particular groups of people (e.g., professors, rock musicians).

Chapter 4: Consensus

Consensus concerns the question of whether two different perceivers of the same target agree about the standing of that target on a trait. As an example, do Zelda and Heidi agree in their perceptions of Carol's intelligence? Even if perceivers agree, this does not necessarily mean that they are accurate.

Consensus is studied for different traits and different levels of acquaintance. Overall, the level of consensus is not very impressive. However, consensus is particularly high for the Big Five factor of Extroversion. Also, consensus for Extroversion occurs very early in the acquaintance process, and there is relatively little change in the rating of a target on that trait. Surprisingly, the research evidence shows that increasing acquaintance does not result in greater consensus. A general model of perception, called the "Weighted-Average Model" (WAM), is developed that explains this surprising finding.

Chapter 5: Uniqueness

Perceivers can have rather idiosyncratic views of a target. In fact, uniqueness is a dominant component in other-perception. Uniqueness effects can be attributed to one of three sources. First, the information that a perceiver uses to judge a target may be different from the information used by other perceivers. For instance, a wife's view of her husband should be relatively unique, because she is likely to have access to information that others do not. Second, two perceivers may see the same behavior, but they may attach different meanings to the same event. Third, a person may apply nonbehavioral information (e.g., his or her liking of the target) in the ratings.

Ironically, it is argued that for very different reasons, both strangers and very close friends are more likely than acquaintances to show uniqueness effects, and so the relationship between acquaintance and uniqueness is complex. Also, uniqueness effects are nearly twice as large for measures of liking than they are for trait ratings.

Chapter 6: Reciprocity and Assumed Reciprocity

Reciprocity can be studied at two different levels: the individual and the dyad. At the individual level, the question is whether someone who sees others as hostile is seen by others as hostile. Except for ratings of the Big Five factor of Agreeableness, there is little or no evidence for reciprocity at the individual level.

At the dyadic level, the question is whether in a relationship, if one person sees his or her partner as hostile, the partner sees him or her as hostile. Reciprocity effects at the dyadic level are generally very weak except for measures of liking: If one person likes the other, often that other person returns the liking. Moreover, liking shows increased dyadic reciprocity with increased acquaintance.

Assumed reciprocity concerns the extent to which people think others see them as they see others. So if Zelda thinks that Heidi is arrogant, does Zelda think that Heidi sees her as arrogant? The answer to this question is that assumed reciprocity for other-perception is virtually non-existent. However, for liking, assumed reciprocity is very high: A person thinks that if he or she likes someone, that person likes him or her back. Unrequited love may exist, but it is usually rather short-lived.

Chapter 7: Target Accuracy

Target accuracy concerns the ability of a perceiver to know the target's actual standing on the trait being rated. It is difficult to measure target accuracy because of the obstacle of ascertaining the person's actual standing on a trait. The most appropriate measure is a behavioral measure, but even behavioral data rely on judgments made by perceivers.

The analysis of the accuracy question requires a partitioning of accuracy into components. Two key types of target accuracy are generalized and dyadic accuracy. Generalized accuracy concerns the ability to predict how a person behaves with others in general, whereas dyadic accuracy concerns the ability to predict how someone behaves with the person who made the predictions.

There has been little research on these fundamental questions. The results from two recent studies that look at people's ability to predict behavior are presented. The first study concerns people's ability to know how much time they spend with particular others. The second, and more interesting, study concerns the validity of judgments about Extroversion made at zero acquaintance. Both studies show that people are quite accurate in their perceptions.

Chapter 8: Meta-Perception

Meta-perception is the perception of another person's perception. It is shown in Chapter 8 that meta-perceptions are surprisingly consistent: People mistakenly assume that nearly everyone sees them in the same way.

Two different types of meta-accuracy are distinguished. Generalized meta-accuracy concerns a person's ability to know how others in general see him or her. Dyadic meta-accuracy concerns people's ability to know who views them positively and who views them negatively. Dyadic meta-accuracy is rather weak, whereas generalized meta-accuracy (given that there is consensus) tends to be rather strong. It is speculated that people use self-theories and self-perception, but not feedback from their partners, to achieve meta-accuracy.

Chapter 9: Self-Perception

The differences between self- and other-perception are highlighted in Chapter 9, and various theories and individual differences concerning self-perception are reviewed. Also, evidence is presented that people engage in self-enhancement: They see themselves as better than others.

Assimilation may be related to self-perception, in that people may assume that others are similar to them. So if Zelda thinks that she is lazy, she may also think that other people are lazy. Alternatively, Zelda may think that if she is lazy, others are not very lazy. At issue is the source of assimilation effects: Do people use themselves as a standard in judging others? The bulk of the evidence seems to support the view that people tend to think that others are similar to them, especially for Agreeableness. Evidence from studies that vary the degree of acquaintance shows that the effects of assumed similarity increase with greater familiarity.

A second issue in self-perception is whether people see a person the way the person sees himself or herself. The answer to this question has important implications for social science theory. According to symbolic interactionists, the self arises from the perceptions that others have. The evidence shows that people do share others' conceptions of them, but it does not seem, at least for college students, that other people generally play an important role in shaping a person's self-conceptions. Rather, the self and other use the same information (the person's behavior), and this is what largely leads to agreement.

If the self and other use similar information, a natural question is the relative validity of self- and other-perception. Evidence is presented that consensual other-perception is often more valid than self-perception. Evidence is also presented that peers agree more with each other in rating a target than they agree with the target's self-rating.

Chapter 10: Concluding Comments

The general topics that cut across the nine basic questions are integrated in Chapter 10. An attempt is made to explain the interrelations among self–other agreement, assumed reciprocity, assumed similarity, and reciprocity. The major techniques used in the book are evaluated. Finally, the links between behavior and perception are explored.

Appendix A

In the first appendix, there is a description of 45 different studies that are used as evidence to answer the nine basic questions of interpersonal perception. Appendix A serves as a general reference for details concerning the studies. Usually, when results from only one or two studies are presented in the text, I restate some details from the study. If, however, the results from many studies are presented, the reader should refer to Appendix A for details.

Appendix B

The second appendix presents the details concerning the statistics that are employed in this book. Most readers will not need to consult this appendix, but it should prove to be useful to those who seek to study interpersonal perception in greater depth. A fairly advanced level of statistical knowledge is required to understand Appendix B, but only an elementary level is needed for the text itself.

Appendix C

The third appendix presents an elaborate mathematical model of perception that includes physical appearance, behavior, and other factors. This model, WAM, is introduced in Chapter 4 and is used throughout the book.

Summary

Person perception can be distinguished from object perception in four important ways. First, person perception is two-sided: Each person is both perceiver and target. Second, in person perception, perceivers attempt to read the minds of targets and engage in what is called "metaperception." Third, in person perception, unlike object perception, there is a close linkage between self- and other-perception. Fourth, in person perception, people, unlike objects, change when they are with different interaction partners. Traditional person perception research employs vignettes, which either do not allow for these possibilities or ignore them when they do occur. That is, traditional vignette research studies person perception as if it were no different from object perception.

Interpersonal perception, the topic of this book, involves studying person perception in a context in which people are interacting. It does not use vignettes; rather, it uses real, interacting people who are both perceiving one another and are wondering how others perceive them.

There are three fundamentally different types of perceptions: other-perception, self-perception, and meta-perception. These three types of perceptions give rise to nine different questions in person perception: assimilation, consensus, uniqueness, reciprocity, target accuracy, assumed reciprocity, meta-accuracy, assumed similarity, and self–other agreement.

The remainder of the book presents a discussion of each of these nine questions. However, before these most interesting questions can be answered, SRM — a general framework that can be used to address the basic questions of interpersonal perception — must be considered.

Notes

1. It is interesting that when people start perceiving objects as people, others begin to think that they may be insane. If a person thinks that a chair is perceiving him or her, or the person thinks that the chair is similar to him or her, most observers would begin to question the person's grasp of reality.

2. Social psychologists also use videotapes, audiotapes, and live confederates to convey information to perceivers. Although information in these media is usually richer than vignettes, they still retain the critical feature of a vignette: the controlled presentation of target information to the perceiver.

Chapter 2

A METHODOLOGY FOR THE STUDY OF INTERPERSONAL PERCEPTION

This chapter presents the Social Relations Model (SRM; Kenny & La Voie, 1984; Malloy & Kenny, 1986), which is used in this book to study interpersonal perception. This model treats interpersonal perception as a two-sided process. It also allows for both meta- and self-perception, and it recognizes that people may change when they interact with multiple partners. SRM is a general model of person, not object, perception.

Although the model is highly statistical, one need not have an advanced understanding of statistics to be able to use it to study interpersonal perception. What follows is a fairly nontechnical account of the model. The details of the statistical formulas are presented elsewhere (Kenny, 1981; Kenny & La Voie, 1984; Warner, Kenny, & Stoto, 1979), as well as in Appendix B.

Introduction to the Social Relations Model

Consider two coworkers, Dave and Mary, who have known each other casually after working together for a few months. Dave and Mary have formed impressions of each other. Each can be asked whether he or she thinks that the other is intelligent, friendly, lazy, and anxious. Consider, for instance, Dave's impression of Mary's intelligence, or $D(M)$ according to the system of notation developed in Chapter 1. It is assumed that Dave believes that Mary is a very intelligent person. The following questions can be asked:

• Does Dave think that all people are intelligent? For instance, Dave may be somewhat dim-witted, and so everybody, compared to him, may seem rather bright. To the extent that some people think individuals are intelligent and other people think that individuals are not intelligent, there is what is called a "perceiver effect."

• Does everybody else think that Mary is smart? If people agree about the standing of a target on a trait, there is what is called a "target effect." The issue is how others typically perceive Mary.

In other formulations of SRM, the term "perceiver" is referred to as "actor," and the term "target" is called "partner." The terms "actor" and "partner" are generic terms that are used in SRM. (These terms are used later in this chapter when behavior is discussed.) Within the specific context of interpersonal perception, the terms "perceiver" and "target" are more appropriate. For affective data, the perceiver effect measures how much of a "liker" the person is, and the target effect measures how popular or likable a person is.

Some way of symbolizing the perceiver and target effects is needed. Both terms involve a theoretical average of the perception of many perceivers or targets. The symbol " ⚲ " is used to denote this average or the typical person. So Dave's perceiver effect is symbolized by $D(\text{⚲})$, which denotes Dave's perception of others in general, and Mary's target effect is symbolized by $\text{⚲}(M)$, which denotes how Mary is viewed by others in general.

Both perceiver effects and target effects are individual-level effects that refer to a person. Neither of these effects is relational. The third component in SRM, called the "relationship effect," is a dyadic effect. It measures how Dave uniquely perceives Mary. Say Dave is secretly in love with Mary, and he is infatuated by her. He may see her as a very intelligent woman, although others do not see her as intelligent and although he does not generally see others as intelligent. Relationship effects emerge after the individual-level effects of perceiver and target are removed. To denote relationship effects, lower-case letters are used. Thus, the relationship effect of Dave toward Mary is symbolized by $d(m)$.

The fourth component in SRM is the "constant effect." It represents the average or mean rating across all perceivers, targets, and relationships. With the notation developed above, the average perception across all targets and perceivers can be symbolized by $\text{⚲}(\text{⚲})$.

To summarize, SRM views perception as the sum of four components: constant, perceiver, target, and relationship. If the relationship component of Dave's perception of Mary is denoted as $d(m)$, then the SRM version of this perception can be written as follows:

$$D(M) = \uparrow(\uparrow) + D(\uparrow) + \uparrow(M) + d(m)$$

That is, Dave's perception of Mary is a function of how people typically see others, or $\uparrow(\uparrow)$; how Dave sees others, or $D(\uparrow)$; how Mary is seen by others, or $\uparrow(M)$; and finally how Dave uniquely sees Mary, or $d(m)$.

Table 2.1 presents the basic components of SRM for other-perception. There are five terms in the model: constant, perceiver, target, relationship, and error. The last of these requires some additional explanation. The relationship component has been defined as the unique perception that Dave has of Mary. However, if Dave's views of others are essentially random, he is uniquely perceiving Mary, but it is not possible to conclude that Dave is *relating* uniquely to Mary. As "relationship" has been defined so far, it contains both relationship and error. A way is needed to separate the relationship effect from error. This can be accomplished by asking Dave how he feels about Mary at two or more times. If he is relating uniquely to Mary, then he should perceive her similarly across the different occasions. If he is responding randomly, then he should respond differently at each time. So, if Dave's view of Mary is obtained on two or more occasions, error can be separated from relationship. Of course, Dave's view of Mary may change over time. So a lack of stability in responding does not always imply a lack of a relationship.

Table 2.2 presents a similar SRM decomposition of meta-perception. For instance, Mary may wonder whether Dave sees her as intelligent, or according to the symbols of Chapter 1, $M(D(M))$.

TABLE 2.1. Components of Other-Perception in SRM

Component	Symbol	Definition
Constant	$\uparrow(\uparrow)$	The average level at which perceivers view targets on the trait
Perceiver	$D(\uparrow)$	The extent to which a perceiver sees targets as high or low on the trait
Target	$\uparrow(M)$	The extent to which a target is seen by perceivers as high or low on the trait
Relationship	$d(m)$	The degree to which a given perceiver sees a given target as high or low on the trait, with perceiver and target effects controlled
Error	—	Chance, inconsistent, or unstable aspects of the rating process

Note. The symbol "$\uparrow$" represents the perceptions or behaviors of a large group of perceivers or targets. Lower-case letters symbolize relationship effects. D and M are two persons.

TABLE 2.2. Components of Meta-Perception in SRM

Component	Symbol	Definition
Constant	$↑(↑(↑))$	The average level at which perceivers think they are viewed by targets on the trait
Perceiver	$M(↑(M))$	The extent to which a perceiver thinks that targets view him or her as high or low on the trait
Target	$↑(D(↑))$	The extent to which a target is seen by perceivers as perceiving others as high or low on the trait
Relationship	$m(d(m))$	The degree to which a perceiver thinks that he or she is seen especially favorably or unfavorably by a target
Error	—	Chance, inconsistent, or unstable aspects of meta-perception

Note. See footnote to Table 2.1 for explanation of symbols.

The perceiver effect in meta-perception, or $M(↑(M))$, represents the extent to which a perceiver thinks that he or she makes the same impression on all of his or her interaction partners. (Again, the symbol $↑$ is used to represent the average of perceptions given or received.) The target effect in meta-perception, or $↑(D(↑))$, represents the extent to which a target is seen as either a harsh or lenient judge of other people. The relationship effect, or $m(d(m))$, represents the extent to which a perceiver thinks that he or she makes an especially favorable or unfavorable impression on a target. The constant effect, or $↑(↑(↑))$, represents the average meta-perception. The full model for the perception that Mary has of Dave's perception of her is as follows:

$$M(D(M)) = ↑(↑(↑)) + M(↑(M)) + ↑(D(↑)) + m(d(m))$$

So if Mary is asked whether she thinks that Dave thinks she is intelligent, a positive perceiver effect would indicate that Mary thinks that others think she is intelligent. A low target effect would indicate that Dave is thought by others to see people as not very intelligent. A positive relationship effect would mean that Mary thinks that Dave views her as especially intelligent. Finally, like other-perceptions, meta-perceptions contain an error component that represents chance, random, and unstable aspects in meta-perceptions.

Self-perceptions cannot be partitioned into perceiver, target, and relationship effects because they are not dyadic measures.[1] However, as shown later in the chapter, a self-perception can be correlated with the perceiver and target effects in other- and meta-perception.

Illustrations

Perceptions of Laziness

In the top portion of Table 2.3 are hypothetical ratings by five people of five other people on the trait of laziness; these ratings can range from 1 ("not lazy") to 9 ("lazy"). For instance, Sam rates Tim, or $S(T)$, an 8 out of 9 on laziness—he sees him as a very lazy person.

One way to gauge whether there are any perceiver effects is to average the ratings of each perceiver across the five targets. These means are presented in the last column of Table 2.3a. It can be seen that Tom views the targets as lazier than do all of the other perceivers, and that Joe views the targets as least lazy. To gauge the target effects, the column means (last row in Table 2.3a) can be examined. Abe is seen as the laziest target, and Cal is seen as the least lazy.

The interest is not in knowing who in the group is seen as lazy, but whether there is any perceiver and target variance in the ratings.

TABLE 2.3. Hypothetical Ratings of Laziness on a 9-Point Scale

a. *Scores and Means*

	Target					
Perceiver	Tim	Abe	Cal	Dan	Jon	Mean[a]
Sam	8	7	2	7	5	5.8
Jim	6	8	3	8	6	6.2
Joe	5	7	1	5	4	4.4
Bob	7	8	4	7	7	6.6
Tom	5	9	5	9	7	7.0
Mean[b]	6.2	7.8	3.0	7.2	5.8	6.0[c]

b. *Relationship Effects*

	Target				
Perceiver	Tim	Abe	Cal	Dan	Jon
Sam	2.0	− .6	− .8	.0	− .6
Jim	− .4	.0	− .2	.6	.0
Joe	.4	.8	− .4	− .6	− .2
Bob	.2	− .4	.4	− .8	.6
Tom	− 2.2	.2	1.0	.8	.2

[a]Mean for each perceiver.
[b]Mean for each target.
[c]Overall mean.

So the presence of target and perceiver effects can be indexed by the variance, or s^2, of the target and perceiver means. The variance of the target means is 3.44, and the variance of the perceiver means is 1.0. The data indicate more target variance than perceiver variance. A variance measure states how different people are from one another on that component. So if a measure has a great deal of perceiver variance, then that demonstrates that the perceivers differ quite a bit from one another on how they see others. The larger the variance, the more people differ from one another on that component.

To estimate the relationship effect, the constant, perceiver, and target effects must be subtracted from the score. Table 2.3b presents the estimates of the relationship effects for the 25 ratings. It can be seen that Sam sees Tim as very lazy, but Tom sees Tim as not very lazy. The variance of the relationship effects is .95. So there is about as much relationship variance as there is perceiver variance, and there is roughly three times as much target variance.[2] The total variance (perceiver plus target plus relationship) is 5.39. Overall, 64% of the variance in the ratings is attibutable to target, about 19% to perceiver, and 18% to relationship.

There are complications and adjustments in the estimation of perceiver and target variances (to be discussed later in this chapter and in Appendix B), but the strategy is basically the same as used for the data in Table 2.3. Estimates of perceiver, target, and relationship effects are computed, and with these estimates the variances are computed.

Variance Partitioning from Three Studies

One major use of SRM is the partitioning of variance. Researchers find or create groups of people, and they ask these people to rate one another. The researchers then determine the proportion of variance that is attributable to perceiver, target, and relationship. Table 2.4 presents the variance partitioning table for three variables. I have chosen an other-perception, a meta-perception, and an affect (liking). For illustrative purposes, I have chosen striking examples; the data from most studies are not so clear-cut.

The first example is taken from an unpublished study (Hallmark & Kenny, 1989). Groups of strangers, each consisting of five to six people, were formed. They sat in a circle, and an experimenter asked each person three different questions about what he or she would do in various situations. For instance, the subjects were asked what they would do if they saw another person cheating on an examination.

TABLE 2.4. Proportion of Variance for Three Variables

Trait	Perceiver	Target	Relationship	Error
Extroversion	.06	.39	.27	.28
Meta-perception	.39	.00	.11	.50
Liking	.19	.07	.50	.24

Note. See text for a description of studies.

After the questions were all asked and answered, the subjects rated one another on a series of traits. The two traits discussed here were "outgoing–reserved" and "talkative–silent." These two measures were treated as indicators of an extroversion construct.

The results (Table 2.4, first row) clearly show that the largest variance component was target variance. Some people were rated as very extroverted, and others were rated as very introverted. There was also a fair amount of variance at the relationship level.

The second example comes from a study conducted in Israel (Shechtman & Kenny, in press). The study involved meta-perceptions of college students. A total of 154 people in 22 human relations groups rated one another on oral communication, human interaction, and leadership; they also provided overall ratings. These four measures served as indicators of a competency construct.

The results (Table 2.4, second row) show that the largest systematic source of variance in meta-perception was perceiver variance. People thought that they made basically the same impression on all of their interaction partners. Interestingly, because there was no target variance in the meta-perceptions, there is no evidence that some people were seen as harsh judges of others and others were seen as lenient judges of their peers.

In the last example (Table 2.4, third row), affect was examined. Levine and Snyder (1980) observed two classes of 5- and 6-year-old children, each 25 in number. Each child rated how much he or she wanted to sit with, work with, and share with the others in the class. These three measures could be treated as replications, and so a separation of relationship and error could be made. It can be seen that the largest portion of variance was at the relationship level. There were rather weak popularity effects, in that the target variance was only 7%. There was some tendency for some children to like others and for others to dislike others, in that there was nearly 20% perceiver variance.

Design and Analysis Considerations

SRM concerns the consistency of perceptions across different targets and perceivers. So to study interpersonal perception within SRM, the person must be observed with multiple partners. If I am to understand how it is that Dave sees Mary, I must know how Dave sees Helen, Jane, and Betty; and I must also know how Frank, Tom, and Peter see Mary. No relationship can be studied in isolation.

In SRM there are two basic designs: "round-robin" and "block" designs. These two designs are illustrated in Table 2.5. In both cases there are six people, numbered from 1 to 6, who are studied. In a round-robin design, each person interacts with or rates everyone in the group. So if the research participants are members of a sorority, in a round-robin design each member would be paired with every other member. As in Table 2.5a, all six people rate the other five members in the group. The " × " indicates a rating, and a " — " indicates missing data. With interpersonal perception data, the " — " is a self-rating and usually would not be missing data. However, it is still set aside for further

TABLE 2.5. Designs Used for SRM

a. *Round-Robin Design*

	Target					
Perceiver	1	2	3	4	5	6
1	—	×	×	×	×	×
2	×	—	×	×	×	×
3	×	×	—	×	×	×
4	×	×	×	—	×	×
5	×	×	×	×	—	×
6	×	×	×	×	×	—

b. *Block Design*

	Target					
Perceiver	1	2	3	4	5	6
1	—	—	—	×	×	×
2	—	—	—	×	×	×
3	—	—	—	×	×	×
4	×	×	×	—	—	—
5	×	×	×	—	—	—
6	×	×	×	—	—	—

analysis. The minimum requirement for the round-robin design is four people.[3]

In a block design, a group of people is broken into two subgroups. Each person then rates everyone else in the other subgroup. As in Table 2.5b, the six people are broken into two subgroups of three people each. The members of the first subgroup, persons 1 through 3, rate the other three people, persons 4 through 6. The minimum requirement for the block design is two people in each subgroup, four people total.

One might wonder why a block design would ever be chosen over a round-robin design. There are two occasions in which a block design is more advantageous than a round-robin design. First, if the researcher wants each subject to interact with other subjects one at a time, a block design requires a minimum of two interaction partners, whereas a round-robin design requires three partners. When there is not sufficient time for three interactions, the block design is preferable. Second, some dyads are asymmetric, in the sense that the two persons are not interchangeable. For example, heterosexual couples are not interchangeable in that the partners can be distinguished by their sex, but gay couples are not asymmetric. Sometimes, when a researcher is interested in asymmetric dyads, certain dyads are not formed. For instance, it would probably be inappropriate to have parents rate other parents or to have men go on "dates" with other men. So for asymmetric dyads, a block design may be more appropriate than a round-robin design.

Sometimes only half the data are gathered from the block design. To return to Table 2.5b, in a "half-block" design, persons 1, 2, and 3 would serve only as perceivers, and persons 4, 5, and 6 would serve only as targets. In such a design, perceptions are not two-sided. A half-block design is typical when the targets are presented on videotape or film.

The block and round-robin designs can also be combined to form a single design. In the block–round-robin design, there are two groups of people, say men and women. In the round-robin part of the design, people rate members of their own sex. In the block part of the design, people rate members of the opposite sex. The block–round-robin design is especially useful for the study of intergroup relations.

There are other designs, as well as variants on the designs that have been described. The reader should consult Kenny (1990) for further elaboration.

The details concerning the statistical analysis of data gathered from SRM designs are presented in Appendix B. Here, I present just a brief introduction to the approach that is taken. This approach can be viewed as a two-way analysis of variance. The two factors are actor or perceiver and partner or target. The model is a random-effects model; that is, the researcher seeks to learn about sources of variation, and not about specific perceivers and targets. To return to Table 2.5, the interest is not in whether target 3 has a high or low target effect, but rather in how much target variance there is.

For a block design, one can obtain perceiver and target variance by using a simple two-way analysis of variance. With a round-robin design, complications arise. The complications concern missing data for the self (the diagonal of the matrix), and some terms are not independent. Appendix B presents solutions to these complications.

Correlations within the Social Relations Model

So far it has been shown how SRM partitions variance into perceiver, target, and relationship components. A second use of the model is to compute correlations. There are two types of correlations: correlations within the same variable, and correlations across two different variables. A correlation within a variable concerns questions of this sort: If Dave likes Mary, does Mary like Dave? Correlations between variables concern questions of this sort: If Dave thinks Mary is attractive, does Dave think that Mary is intelligent?

Correlations within a Variable: Reciprocity

One useful purpose of SRM is that it allows researchers to measure reciprocity. To return to Dave and Mary, this question can be asked: If Dave thinks that Mary is intelligent, or $D(M)$, does Mary think that Dave is intelligent, or $M(D)$? Are their perceptions mirror images of each other? Sometimes perceptions are complementary: Dave thinks that Mary is intelligent, but Mary thinks that Dave is stupid.

Within SRM, there are two types of reciprocity. First, there is "dyadic reciprocity," or reciprocity at the dyadic level. Dave's relationship effect toward Mary is correlated with Mary's relationship effect toward Dave. This is symbolized by $d(m) = m(d)$. Second, there is "generalized reciprocity," or reciprocity at the individual level. For example, Dave's perceiver effect, or $D(\ast)$, may be correlated with his target effect, or $\ast(D)$. So it can be asked whether a person who tends to see others as intelligent tends to be seen by others as intelligent. This correlation is referred to as the "perceiver–target" correlation, and assesses generalized reciprocity. It is symbolized by $D(\ast) = \ast(D)$.

Correlations across Variables

Within SRM, there is often an interest in the correlation between a pair of variables. For instance, the pair of variables may be other-perceptions of intelligence and meta-perceptions of intelligence. Surprisingly, there are six, not one, possible correlations between the two variables: four correlations can be computed at the individual level, and two at the dyadic level. Individual-level correlations involve the perceiver and target effects of SRM, and dyadic-level correlations involve the relationship effect.

Individual Level

The four types of correlations between components at the individual level are "perceiver–perceiver," "perceiver–target," "target–perceiver," and "target–target." To follow the text more easily, readers will probably find it helpful to consult Tables 2.1 and 2.2. It is also helpful to realize that the symbol for the perceiver effect for Dave is $D(\nearrow)$, and that the symbol for the target effect is $\nearrow(D)$. The four individual-level correlations are defined as follows in terms of Dave's other- and meta-perceptions of intelligence:

> Perceiver–perceiver: $D(\nearrow) = D(\nearrow(D))$. If D sees others as intelligent, does D think that others see him as intelligent?
> Perceiver–target: $D(\nearrow) = \nearrow(D(\nearrow))$. If D sees others as intelligent, do others think that D sees them as intelligent?
> Target–perceiver: $\nearrow(D) = D(\nearrow(D))$. If D is seen by others as intelligent, does D think that others see him as intelligent?
> Target–target: $\nearrow(D) = \nearrow(D(\nearrow))$. If D is seen by others as intelligent, do others think that D sees them as intelligent?

As discussed later in this chapter, the middle two correlations assess meta-accuracy, and the first and last assess assumed reciprocity.

Dyadic Level

There are two types of correlations between relationship components: "intrapersonal" and "interpersonal" relationship correlations. These two correlations between other- and meta-perceptions of intelligence between Dave and Mary are as follows:

> Intrapersonal: $d(m) = d(m(d))$. If D thinks that M is especially intelligent, does D think that M sees him as especially intelligent?

Interpersonal: $d(m) = m(d(m))$. If D thinks that M is especially intelligent, does M think that D sees her as especially intelligent?

As seen later, the first question assesses assumed reciprocity at the dyadic level, whereas the second assesses meta-accuracy.

The first question is called "intrapersonal" because it concerns two thoughts that the same person (Dave) has about another (Mary). The second is called "interpersonal" because it concerns the association between the thought that a person has about another, and the latter person's thought about the former person. Thus, in an interpersonal correlation the thoughts of two different people are correlated, whereas in an intrapersonal correlation the thoughts of the same person are correlated.

The Social Relations Model and Interpersonal Perception

I now consider the partitioning of other- and meta-perception into components of SRM. Chapter 1 has presented nine fundamental questions in interpersonal perception. In this section, I show how these questions can be answered by using SRM. A summary of this section is presented in Table 2.6. This introductory presentation of the use of SRM to answer the nine fundamental questions is rather abstract; the questions are discussed in more concrete detail in subsequent chapters.

The question of assimilation concerns variance in the perceiver effect, or $D(\uparrow)$. If some perceivers tend to view targets favorably and others tend to see targets unfavorably, then there is perceiver variance. Assimilation is measured by the amount of perceiver variance. Typically, what is computed is the relative amount of perceiver variance — the perceiver variance divided by the sum of all sources of variance. If the symbols stand for variance, assimilation is indexed by $D(\uparrow)/[D(\uparrow) + \uparrow(D) + d(m)]$.

The question of consensus concerns variance in the target effect, or $\uparrow(D)$. If perceivers agree about the standing of targets on a trait, then there is target variance. As with assimilation effects, the relative target variance is typically computed — the target variance divided by the total variance. If the symbols stand for variance, consensus is indexed by $\uparrow(D)/[D(\uparrow) + \uparrow(D) + d(m)]$.

The question of uniqueness concerns variance in the relationship effect, or $d(m)$. If interpersonal perception is unique, then relationship variance can index that phenomenon. Often the relative relationship variance is computed — relationship variance divided by the total

TABLE 2.6. Expression of Basic Questions Using SRM

Effect	Level	Symbol
Assimilation	Individual	$D(\text{🧍})$
Consensus	Individual	$\text{🧍}(D)$
Uniqueness	Dyadic	$d(m)$
Reciprocity	Individual	$D(\text{🧍}) = \text{🧍}(D)$
	Dyadic	$d(m) = m(d)$
Target accuracy	Individual	$M(\text{🧍}) = \text{🧍}_M$
	Individual	$\text{🧍}(D) = D_{\text{🧍}}$
	Dyadic	$m(d) = d_m$
Assumed reciprocity	Individual	$D(\text{🧍}) = D(\text{🧍}(D))$
	Individual	$\text{🧍}(M) = \text{🧍}(M(\text{🧍}))$
	Dyadic	$d(m) = d(m(d))$
Meta-accuracy	Individual	$\text{🧍}(D) = D(\text{🧍}(D))$
	Individual	$M(\text{🧍}) = \text{🧍}(M(\text{🧍}))$
	Dyadic	$m(d) = d(m(d))$
Assumed similarity	Individual	$D(D) = D(\text{🧍})$
Self–other agreement	Indivdual	$D(D) = \text{🧍}(D)$

Note. See footnote to Table 2.1 for explanation of symbols.

variance. To have a valid measure of uniqueness, there should be multiple measures of the variable. If there are not, then relationship variance also contains error variance.

Reciprocity occurs at two levels. At the individual level, it is the perceiver–target correlation, or $D(\text{🧍}) = \text{🧍}(D)$. If some people see all targets as intelligent, are these people seen by others as intelligent? At the dyadic level, the reciprocity correlation is between relationship effects: $d(m) = m(d)$. If Dave sees Mary as particularly intelligent, does Mary see Dave as particularly intelligent? Both are correlations within a variable. The correlations to be discussed for the remaining five questions are across different variables.

Target accuracy is the degree of correspondence between a person's perception of a target person with that target's actual standing on the trait or D. The measurement of target accuracy depends on how the person's actual standing on the trait is measured. If the measure of actual standing is a single, global measure, then target accuracy is indexed by the correlation of the target effect in other-perception with the target's actual standing, or $\text{🧍}(D) = D$.

However, the measure of a person's behavior may change for different interaction partners. A person may be cooperative with one person but not with another. If the target's behavior changes across interaction partners, the variance of the behavior can be partitioned into three sources: actor, partner, and relationship. The actor effect for Dave is denoted as $D_{\uparrow}$; the partner effect for Mary is denoted as $\uparrow_M$; and how Dave particularly behaves when he is with Mary is denoted as d_m. The actor effect, or $D_{\uparrow}$, represents how the person behaves across all of his or her interaction partners. So, for example, is Dave cooperative with all of his interaction partners? The partner effect, or $\uparrow_M$, assesses the behavior that a person consistently elicits from others. So are people cooperative when they interact with Mary? Finally, the relationship effect, or d_m, measures the way a person uniquely behaves with a given partner. So is Dave particularly cooperative when he interacts with Mary?

Each of these three components of behavior can be correlated with Mary's perception of Dave's level of cooperation. There are three different measures of target accuracy. The target–actor correlation, or $\uparrow(D) = D_{\uparrow}$, assesses whether Dave, who is seen as cooperative by others, acts cooperatively with all of his interaction partners. The perceiver–partner correlation, or $M(\uparrow) = \uparrow_M$, assesses the extent to which Mary, who sees others as cooperative, elicits cooperative behavior from others. Finally, the relationship correlation, or $m(d) = d_m$, assesses whether Mary, who sees Dave as especially cooperative, is correct in predicting Dave's level of cooperation when interacting with Mary.

Assumed reciprocity can be measured in three ways: two at the individual level, and one at the dyadic level. The first measure of assumed reciprocity at the individual level is the correlation between the perceiver effect in other-perception and the perceiver effect in reflected appraisal or meta-perception, or $D(\uparrow) = D(\uparrow(D))$. If Dave sees others as intelligent, does he think that others see him as intelligent? The second measure at the individual level is the correlation between the target effect in other-perception and the target effect in meta-perception, or $\uparrow(M) = \uparrow(M(\uparrow))$: If Mary is seen as intelligent, do people assume that she sees others as intelligent? The final assumed-reciprocity correlation is between relationship effects, or $d(m) = d(m(d))$. If Dave sees Mary as especially intelligent, does Dave think that Mary sees him as especially intelligent?

Meta-accuracy, like assumed reciprocity, is indexed by three different correlations. The first correlation at the individual level is the correlation between the target effect in other-perception and the perceiver effect in meta-perception, or $\uparrow(D) = D(\uparrow(D))$. If Dave is seen as intelligent by others, does Dave think that others see him as intelligent? The second correlation is the correlation between the perceiver effect in other-perception and the target effect in meta-perception, or $M(\uparrow) = \uparrow(M(\uparrow))$. If Mary thinks that other people are intelligent, do others know that Mary sees people that way? The third correlation is at the level of the relationship, or $m(d) = d(m(d))$. If Mary sees Dave as particularly intelligent, does Dave know that Mary sees him that way?

Assumed similarity is the correspondence between the perceiver effect in other-perception and the self-perception, or $D(D) = D(\textnormal{\textdagger})$. If Dave thinks that he is intelligent, does he think that others are also intelligent? Self–other agreement is the correspondence between the target effect in other-perception with self-perception, or $D(D) = \textnormal{\textdagger}(D)$. If Dave sees himself as intelligent, do others also see him as intelligent?

Basic Statistics

Generally in the social sciences, the basic statistics that are reported are means. In this book, they are variances and correlations. Moreover, many variances and correlations that are reported in this book are derived and not directly computed variances and correlations. In this section, I describe these statistics so that they can be more easily understood when they are presented in subsequent chapters.

Variance

It is helpful to return to the example in Table 2.3. Recall that in this example, five people rate how lazy five different people are. To measure the target effect, the ratings of each target are averaged across the five perceivers. The measure of target variance is the variance of target means, which equals 3.44 for the data in Table 2.3a.

The amount of variance in the target means depends on the number of perceivers over which the means are averaged. The greater the number of perceivers, the smaller the variance. For instance, if there were just two perceivers in Table 2.3 (i.e., if three were randomly discarded), the target variance would increase to 3.725, an 8% increase. So the amount of variance in the target means depends on the number of perceivers that are used to compute the target means. Similarly, the variance in the perceiver means depends on the number of targets.

Most researchers would prefer that the measure of target variance not depend on the number of perceivers. The strategy within SRM is to forecast what the target variance would be if there were many perceivers. This is accomplished by taking the variance of the targets and subtracting a correction term that is based on the number of perceivers and the relationship variance. (See Appendix B for the exact formulas.) So for instance, for the data in Table 2.3a the variance in the target means is 3.44, but the forecast of target variance, if there were an infinite number of perceivers, is 3.25.

Consider what would happen if, to give another example, there were no target variance. There would still be variance in the target means, because people's perceptions would depend on the specific relationships that they had formed. So if there were ratings of intelligence and the targets did not differ in their perceived intelligence, some targets would appear a bit more intelligent than others, because they just happened to be rated by persons whose relationship effects toward them were positive. If the target means were computed across more perceivers, there would be less variance. If there were an infinite number of perceivers, the variance in the target means would be zero. Of course, it is impossible to measure the target variance with an infinite number of perceivers. So within SRM, the perceiver and target variances are the best guesses of what the variance would be if there were an infinite number of perceivers. Thus, the estimate of target variance is a theoretical variance and not an actual variance of scores.

Because both the target and perceiver variances are theoretical extrapolations, they can be estimated as negative. If the true target variance were very small, then about half the time it would be estimated as negative. Negative variances, though impossible when using the ordinary formulas for variance, are possible in the computation of theoretical variances. When the variances are computed as negative, it is a common practice to report them as zero. Negative variances are quite anomalous, but they are the price that is paid to ensure that target variances do not depend on the number of perceivers and that perceiver variances do not depend on the number of targets.

Generally, as in Table 2.4, this text presents relative variances. For instance, the relative perceiver variance is the perceiver variance divided by the sum of all the variances in the model. A relative variance can be interpreted as if it were a correlation. For instance, the relative target variance is the predicted correlation between pairs of different raters judging the same set of targets. So, for instance, if there were 20 perceivers and 10 targets and each target was judged by two different perceivers, the relative target variance would be the correlation between the two targets' judgments.[4]

Similar adjustments are made to the variances when multiple measures are used. Recall that for the relationship variance to be separated from error, the perceiver must rate the target twice. Within SRM, if there are multiple measures, a variance is the best guess of what the variance would be if scores were averaged over an infinite number of measures.

Correlation

A correlation is a measure of linear association between a pair of variables. For a positive correlation, as one variable increases, so does the other. For instance, as children get older, they get taller, and so age and height are positively correlated. A negative correlation implies that as one variable increases, the other decreases. For instance, as an adult man gets older, he often has less hair.

The preceding section has shown how having a finite number of perceivers artificially increases the variance in the target means. Within SRM, the variances are forecasts of what they would be if there were a large number of perceivers or targets.

Variances are used in computing correlations: The correlation between variables X and Y is defined as the covariance between X and Y divided by the square root of the product of the variances of X and Y. (The covariance between X and Y is defined as $\Sigma(X - M_X)(Y - M_Y)/(n - 1)$.) Within SRM, the actual variances are not used, but the theoretical variances are used. The resulting correlation is said to be "corrected for attenuation." Because the correlations are divided by something smaller, the resulting correlations are larger than they would be if they were not corrected for attenuation.

The ordinary correlations are smaller than they should be because people interact with a finite number of partners or the number of measures is finite. A correlation that is corrected for attenuation removes the artificial lowering of the correlation that results from the finite number of partners or measures. To express these disattenuated correlations and distinguish them from attenuated correlations, they are printed in this book in italics. So, for instance, .2 is used to represent an ordinary correlation, and *.2* is used to represent a disattenuated correlation.

Also, many correlations within SRM are derived correlations. That is, the correlations have been mathematically adjusted for other correlations. For instance, the perceiver–target correlation is not the simple correlation because the dyadic-reciprocity correlation is adjusted from it. Given that a correlation is derived, it can be larger than 1 or smaller than −1. The usual convention is followed by setting the out-of-range correlations to +1 if they are positive and to −1 if they are negative.

Significance Tests

Most of the results that are presented in this book are correlations. Recall that relative perceiver and target variances can be interpreted as correlation coefficients. Unfortunately, these correlations cannot be tested in the usual way, because they use adjusted variances in their estimation. Significance testing within SRM is described in Appendix B. When presenting correlations and relative variances, I do not report whether the correlations are significant or not. If I were to report statistical significance, tables would be needlessly cluttered, and the reader would be distracted in trying to figure out why some correlations are significant and others are not. The reader should pay attention to the size of the correlations and the pattern.

Summary

The study of interpersonal perception requires a different research paradigm. The experimental paradigm in which artificially constructed targets are presented to perceivers is not well suited to answer the basic questions of interpersonal perception posed in Chapter 1. SRM, however, is ideally suited to the study of person perception in an interpersonal context.

SRM partitions other-perception data into three major sources of variance: perceiver, target, and relationship. The perceiver effect represents how the perceiver generally sees others; the target effect represents how the target is generally seen by others; and the relationship effect represents how a person uniquely sees a given target.

Specific designs in which each perceiver rates multiple targets and each target is judged by multiple perceivers are required to estimate the parameters of SRM. To separate error from relationship, there must be multiple measures of the theoretical construct. The parameters of SRM can be estimated by a variant of two-way random-effects analysis of variance: perceiver and target.

The nine basic questions can be answered by using SRM. Three of the nine questions are answered using variances, one by a correlation within a variable, and the remaining five by correlations between variables. Many questions can be addressed at both the individual and the dyadic levels.

The basic statistics to be presented in this text are variances and correlations. The interpretation of these measures is discussed. It is pointed out that sometimes these values can be out of range; that is, variances can be negative, and correlations can be greater than 1. Although these anomalous values are not possible with ordinary variances and correlations, they happen within SRM because estimates are forecasts of variances and correlations based on an infinite number of perceivers, targets, and measures.

The stage is now set. The remaining chapters present the fascinating investigation into the nine basic questions of interpersonal perception.

Notes

1. Error or unstable variance can be removed if there are multiple measures.

2. The relationship variance is defined as the sum of the relationship effects squared, divided by the number of perceivers minus 1 times the number of targets minus 1.

3. If it can be assumed that there is no dyadic reciprocity, then the group size can be as small as three.

4. If the same perceivers rated all of the targets, that correlation would be estimated by the ratio of target variance to the sum of target plus relationship variance.

Chapter 3

ASSIMILATION

"**A**ssimilation" concerns the basic question of whether the same perceiver sees two targets in essentially the same way. More colloquially, the assimilation question is "Do they all look alike?" If each perceiver were to give exactly the same rating to all targets, and the perceivers were to differ from one another in their ratings, assimilation effects would be at their highest. However, normally there is not perfect assimilation; at issue is the extent to which perceivers assimilate targets. As seen in Chapter 2, assimilation effects can be assessed by the amount of perceiver variance in the Social Relations Model (SRM). Note that assimilation refers to the *variance* in the perceiver effect. If all perceivers see the targets in the same way, there is no perceiver variance, and consequently there is no assimilation.[1]

It seems obvious that people differ in the standards that they set for themselves in evaluating others. Some people expect the best from others, and these perceivers seem never to be satisfied. Professor Kingsfield, the fictional law professor in the movie and television series *The Paper Chase,* for example, holds particularly high expectations for others. For other perceivers, even the smallest level of a behavior is enough. An example of a perceiver who sees the best in people is Fred Rogers of the *Mister Rogers' Neighborhood* television show for preschoolers.

It seems obvious that some perceivers are harsh and others are lenient, but the explanation of these differences is not so obvious. There are three major explanations of assimilation. In the first, assimilation is viewed as a methodological artifact; that is, assimilation reflects a response style and has no psychological meaning. In the second explanation, the perceiver effect reflects the perceiver's view of the generalized other; that is, the perceiver effect reflects how the person thinks people are in general. In the third explanation, the perceiver effect reflects the perceiver's view of the typical other in the group. That is, the perceiver effect reflects not a general view of how others are in general, but rather a more local view of how others are in a particular group. These three different explanations of assimilation are considered in turn.

The Response Set Interpretation of Assimilation

The first explanation is purely methodological, although not very interesting. It is possible that assimilation may not reflect any psychological process, but may be only a function of how the perceiver assigns numbers to targets. For instance, some perceivers may routinely use large numbers in rating targets, whereas other perceivers may use relatively small numbers. The perceivers' reasons for doing so may reflect nothing very interesting psychologically, but only a measurement bias.

Psychometricians have used the term "response set" to refer to a tendency for the responses of perceivers to reflect a response pattern and not something psychological. Whenever one analyzes rating data, it is important to realize that response set may be a factor.

Research Evidence

Perhaps because this explanation is methodological and not very exciting, there has been little concerted effort to test the extent to which perceiver effects in interpersonal perception measure something more than response set. One important study was conducted by Crow and Hammond (1957, Study 2). They studied 72 medical students at the University of Colorado at three times: the beginning, middle, and end of the academic year. At each time point, the medical students rated a different set of 10 patients. Crow and Hammond found that those medical students who rated targets very favorably at one time also rated a different set of targets very favorably at the other two times. And those who rated targets unfavorably at the first time tended to rate the targets very unfavorably at the next two times. Recall that different targets were being rated at each time. This study thus indicates that there is assimilation, but does not indicate its source.

One way to determine whether response set is the only determinant of perceiver effects is to compute the correlation of perceiver effects across measures of different traits. If the perceiver correlation between the ratings of two traits (e.g., between perceivers' average ratings of intelligence and friendliness) is near 1, then that would be supportive of the response set interpretation. If the correlation is less than 1, then the nonoverlapping variance would be an indication that the perceiver effect changes from trait to trait—something that is more difficult to explain purely in terms of response sets. It is important in carrying out such an analysis to make certain that the traits are conceptually distinct, so that they do not correlate because of content overlap.

Such an analysis can be performed using data from a study (Albright, Kenny, & Malloy, 1988, Study 3) in which perceivers rated five independent personality traits in a situation in which the targets were strangers. People rated three, four, or five other people on numbered 7-point scales on the traits "sociable," "good-natured," "responsible," "calm," and "intellectual." The correlation of perceiver effects between pairs of traits was .55. This means that about half the perceiver variance[2] was stable from trait to trait. So it seems that it is not true that the tendency to use a particular part of the scale is the whole story for perceiver effects. Note that the .55 correlation is a disattenuated correlation (see Chapter 2), and so it is larger than an ordinary product–moment correlation between the perceiver effects of the two traits.

A second study that can be used to evaluate the unidimensionality of perceiver effects is that of Dantchik (1985). This study examined the ratings of targets who were members of the same sorority or fraternity, and so the perceivers and targets were relatively well acquainted. There were six traits: intelligence, likability, self-control, sociability, adjustment, and dominance. The average perceiver–perceiver correlation among the six factors was .51. So, as with the unacquainted people, there is a substantial but not a perfect correlation between the perceiver effects of traits.

The perceiver effect seems to have two different parts. There is a global, undifferentiated view of what the group members are like; this global part probably mainly consists of response set. Then there is a more differentiated view. This second component is probably not response set, but rather reflects real differences that the perceiver sees in all the targets on different traits. These two components of the perceiver effect correspond closely, but not identically, to two components of ratings posited by Cronbach (1955). He referred to the general view of others' standing on all the traits as "elevation," and he referred to how the targets differ on the traits as "stereotype." It seems that these two components, elevation and stereotype, explain about the same amount of variance.

A second way to evaluate the response set hypothesis is to reverse the traits. The rating instrument is designed in the following fashion: For about half the traits, the larger numbers indicate more positive standing on the traits, and for the remaining traits, the smaller numbers indicate more positive standing. If numbers are not used, but rather the perceiver checks a box, then for half the scales the positive end is on the right side of the page, and for the other half the positive end is placed on the left side of the page.

At issue is the effect of reversal on the perceiver–perceiver correlation between the positive and negative traits. A correlation of *1.00* would indicate that response set is the tendency to use higher or lower numbers (or, if check marks are used, the tendency to respond on the left or right side of the page). However, a correlation near *– 1.00* would indicate that response set reflects the general impression that the perceiver has toward all the targets—that is, the tendency for the perceiver to view favorably or unfavorably all the targets in the group. As earlier discussed, the perceiver effect contains two components, each explaining about 50% of the variance. The correlations that are now considered are those from the general or common part of the perceiver effect, which is more likely to correspond to the response set.

Results from three different studies are examined. The first is a study (Albright et al., 1988, Study 1) that used the zero-acquaintance paradigm. As discussed in Chapter 1, in this paradigm perceivers observe the targets but do not interact with them. People rated one another on five scales, two of which were reversed. The correlation between the reversed and unreversed perceiver effects was *– .87.* This supports the view that perceiver effect reflects, in large part, the perceiver's overall *evaluation* of the targets.

The remaining two studies used check marks and not numerical ratings. These two studies also support the general-impression view of perceiver effects. The correlation from one study (Study 2 from Kenny, Horner, Kashy, & Chu, 1992) was *– 1.00,* and that from the other (Levesque, 1990) was *– .94.* Perceiver variance seems largely to reflect how a person generally views members of that group.

In conclusion, it appears that there is a single variable that determines about half the variance in the perceiver effect for ratings of targets. However, this variable is not a pure measurement artifact. It seems to reflect how the perceiver evaluates the targets in the group; that is, it reflects how much the perceiver likes the people in the group. Thus, the pure response set interpretation receives little or no support.[3] Moreover, evidence presented later in this chapter on stereotypes provides additional evidence that the perceiver effect represents something psychologically meaningful.

Design Considerations

There are ways of gathering data that may reduce or even eliminate the response set problem. One approach is to vary the rating format.

Research (Guilford, 1954, pp. 263–269) indicates that it is preferable to use blanks and not numbers. So, for instance, if the rating is on the dimension "active–passive," the rating form would look like this—

Active |___|___|___|___|___|___|___| Passive

instead of this:

Active   1   2   3   4   5   6   7   Passive

The use of check marks seems to reduce the amount of response set.[4]

Another possible procedure to reduce response set is to have perceivers rate one target at a time on all the traits, as opposed to having perceivers rate all the targets on each trait before moving on to the next trait. A colleague and I (Hallmark & Kenny, 1989) conducted a study to evaluate the effect of rating format on the amount of perceiver variance. Our prediction was that having perceivers rate one target at a time would increase the amount of perceiver variance across traits. Quite surprisingly, there were no differences between the two different types of rating formats. Some evidence even pointed to the superiority of the person format approach (i.e., rating each target on all the traits before moving on to the next target) over the trait format.

One way to eliminate the problem of response set is to ask the perceivers to rank-order the targets. For example, if there are eight targets, the perceivers assign numbers from 1 to 8 to the targets. Such a procedure totally eliminates the perceiver effect. One study (Zaccaro, Foti, & Kenny, 1991) compared rankings and ratings of leadership in three-person groups. The correlation of the extent to which the target was seen as a leader using rankings and ratings was .98. Another study (Chapdelaine, Kenny, & LaFontana, in press) used rankings versus ratings to examine liking. The research participants were groups of five women who interacted one-on-one. That study found a perfect correlation between the target effects of the two methods. Thus, there is little or no difference between the two measurement methods. However, because the group size was only three in one study and five in the other, it is not known whether rankings and ratings would be essentially equivalent with larger group sizes.[5]

The use of rankings eliminates the perceiver effect, and so it is impossible to measure assimilation effects. So rankings should only be employed if a researcher has no interest in the perceiver effect. Ranking forces perceivers to make discriminations between targets that may not really exist. Also, with many targets, ranking is a very burdensome procedure.

Sometimes researchers force perceivers to use a particular distribution in making their ratings. The Q-sort method (Nunnally, 1967), one such procedure, forces the perceiver to form a quasi-normal distribution of responses. Like ranking, the Q-sort eliminates the perceiver effect.

Response set seems more likely to intrude into ratings when subjects have little or no motivation to respond carefully. Whenever possible, it is important to reduce the burden on subjects by not giving them page after page of ratings. If extensive ratings must be made, then investigators should provide both incentives to increase the subjects' motivation and rest periods.

Stereotype Interpretations of Assimilation

The Generalized-Other Interpretation

Apparently there is evidence that a good deal of variance in perceiver effects reflects something beyond a measurement artifact. Recall that one early piece of evidence for assimilation was the study by Crow and Hammond (1957), which showed that medical students consistently differed in how they viewed their patients. Some viewed patients very negatively, whereas others viewed patients very positively. These doctors-to-be differed in their patient stereotypes.

The second interpretation of the perceiver effect is that it reflects a view of how a person sees other people in general. According to this view, people carry around in their heads a view of what the typical other person is like. Within this framework, the perceiver effect reflects people's phenomenology; that is, it reflects how people view their world.

According to this view, the perceiver effect reflects a stereotype—a set of assumptions that a person makes about others. It is important to realize that these stereotypes, unlike racial and gender stereotypes, differ across perceivers. Some perceivers have positive views of others, whereas other perceivers have negative views of others.

Over the years, numerous psychologists have proposed that people view the world with a general expectancy about others. The personality psychologist George Kelly (1955) referred to "personal constructs," which are central dimensions on which people evaluate others. The social psychologists Higgins and Bargh (1987) have used the term "chronicity" to describe people's repeated use of the same dimension in evaluating others. Markus (1977) has proposed the related construct of being "schematic" versus "aschematic" on a trait. As an example of these concepts, it would seem that professors tend to use the dimension of intelligence in evaluating others. Over three decades ago, Bronfenbrenner, Harding, and Gallwey (1958) suggested the term "generalized other," which was initially put forth in another context (see Chapter 8) by the philosopher George Herbert Mead (1934). The generalized other (the term to be used in this chapter) reflects a person's view of human nature.

The view of the typical other may change, depending on the rating context.[6] First, there is people's view of what others are like. Second, there is people's view of what others are like when they interact with them. So a man may think that others are friendly and nice, but he may also believe that when people interact with him, they are hostile.

Although it seems plausible that people's view of others in general and their view of others interacting with them may differ, there is little evidence concerning the difference between these two types of perceiver effects. In one study that did investigate the stability of the perceiver effect in dyadic and group interactions (Study 2 of Kenny et al., 1992), the perceiver effect was measured during zero acquaintance and during a one-on-one interaction. Interestingly, the one factor of the Big Five (see Chapter 1) that showed the weakest correlation across situations was Agreeableness. So people who viewed others as agreeable did not necessarily see them as very agreeable when they interacted with them. The perceiver effect may be very different in the perception of partners in dyadic interactions ("how others are with me") and in the general perception of others ("how others behave in general").

Assimilation and Acquaintance

The stereotype explanation of the perceiver effect is that one person views another without any information. Therefore, the perceiver effect reflects the perceiver's ignorance. That is, it is a guess about what the typical other person is like. Presumably, as more information becomes available, this expectancy would be used less. So if Sally thought that others were generally friendly and warm, she would rate others that way, but once she got to know them, she would rely less on her stereotype (Locksley, Borgida, Brekke, & Hepburn, 1980). In this context, I review three studies that examined changes in perceiver variance over time and one study that compared the ratings of friends and acquaintances.

The first two studies examined the transition from zero acquaintance to acquaintance based on social interaction. In both studies, people rated one another in face-to-face noninteractive settings, and then interacted. In one of these studies (Kenny et al., 1992, Study 2), the interactions were one-on-one; in the other (Albright et al., 1988, Study 1), the interactions were in a classroom situation. In the Albright et al. study, the students were remeasured at midsemester (wave 1) and at the end of the semester (wave 2).

Table 3.1 presents the *absolute* amount of perceiver variance on each of the Big Five factors for both studies. It seems fairly clear that the level of perceiver variance declined from the zero acquaintance situation to the actual interaction situation. All five of the variances declined in the Kenny et al. study, and 7 of the 10 comparisons declined in the Albright et al. study. Moreover, two of the increases are attributable to the especially low levels of perceiver variance at zero acquaintance for the Emotional Stability factor in this study. From these results, it seems reasonable to conclude that perceiver variance does indeed decline as a function of acquaintance.

The Albright et al. study can also be used to evaluate the decline in assimilation as a function of acquaintance for those who were more than minimally acquainted with the targets. In all five comparisons, there was a decline in perceiver variance. Similar declines can also be seen in Study 1 of the Park and Judd (1989) study, although for some unknown reason assimilation effects appeared to rebound at the last session.

The rate of decline in these studies is rather substantial. For the two studies that used zero acquaintance as a baseline (Albright et al.

TABLE 3.1. Absolute Perceiver Variance as a Function of Acquaintance

Kenny, Horner, Kashy, & Chu (1992), Study 2

	Wave 0	Wave 1
Extroversion	.273	.068
Agreeableness	.250	.120
Conscientiousness	.497	.256
Emotional Stability	.386	.363
Culture	.380	.216

Albright, Kenny, & Malloy (1988), Study 1

	Wave 0	Wave 1	Wave 2
Extroversion	.254	.082	.009
Agreeableness	.420	.781	.253
Conscientiousness	.403	.265	.130
Emotional Stability	.145	.478	.313
Culture	.477	.314	.146

Park & Judd (1989), Study 1

	Wave 1	Wave 2	Wave 3	Wave 4
Median of 17 traits	.358	.339	.213	.276

and Kenny et al.), about 54% of the initial perceiver variance persisted. For the Park and Judd study of increasing acquaintance, about 77% of the variance persisted. These declines are even more impressive when one realizes that about 50% of the variance is attributable to response set, and that it is likely that response set variance does not decline.

A further test of the hypothesis that assimilation declines as acquaintance increases can be performed using the data from a study (Kenny & Kashy, in press) in which we compared the perceptions of friends versus acquaintances. If assimilation is more prevalent when less is known about the target, there should be less perceiver variance in the ratings of friends than in those of acquaintances. For three of the four variables examined in this study, there was less perceiver variance in the ratings of friends versus acquaintances; across the four variables, the friend-to-acquaintance ratio in perceiver variance was .86. Thus, this study provides some support for the claim that assimilation declines with increasing acquaintance.

Across all the studies, it can be concluded that assimilation effects do decline as a function of acquaintance. Perceivers draw more heavily on their stereotype of the generalized other when they know little or nothing about the targets, but as they begin to know more about the targets, there is less assimilation. This seems especially true during the early stages of acquaintance.

Origins of the Generalized Other

There are two alternate theories concerning how a person's view of the generalized other is formed. The first view is that the perceiver effect reflects how a person sees himself or herself. The second view is that the perceiver effect reflects the person's view of significant others—in particular, the person's parents or close friends.

Self. The view that how one sees others is related to how one sees oneself is the question of assumed similarity, which is a central focus in Chapter 9. It is also considered in Chapter 6 when the projection hypothesis is considered. Projection differs from assumed similarity as follows: In projection, perceivers see others as the perceivers *really* are, whereas in assumed similarity, perceivers see others as the perceivers themselves *think* they are.

But there is a less obvious way in which the perceiver effect may reflect self-perception—one that is quite different from both assumed similarity and projection: The self can be used to anchor the scale. If it is believed that people see themselves as average or typical (see Chapter 9 for a different view), they should put themselves at the midpoint of the scale. So if a 7-point scale were used, they would give themselves a rating of 4. If self is used as an anchor, then people should be rating others in relation to their self-perceptions. Thus, if one person were to see himself or herself as fairly high on a trait, that person would see most others as lower than him or her, and so would give them low numbers. Alternatively, if the person were to see himself or herself as low on the scale, he or she would view others favorably. Given this perspective, the perceiver effect would reflect the person's self-perception on the dimension being rated, but the perceiver effect would correlate negatively with the person's self-perception. It would seem that this hypothesis would be more likely for ratings of ability than of personality.

One might argue that the model underlying the predicted negative self-perceiver correlation is invalid, because when people rate themselves on a scale, they rarely place themselves at the scale midpoint; rather, they typically place themselves above the scale midpoint (see Chapter 9). However, because self-ratings are often distorted by self-presentational processes, they may not adequately reflect the person's true self-perception. One might make the bold argument that self-perception may be best measured by the perceiver effect and not directly by the self-rating.

Another argument against this hypothesis is that it would imply a negative correlation between self-rating and perceiver effect, but (as is seen in Chapter 9) the perceiver–self correlation is usually positive. However (as discussed in Chapter 10), the presence of response set in both the perceiver effect and the self-rating may bring about an artificially positive correlation between the two.

Significant Others.   The view that the generalized other reflects how the person sees significant others has its roots in clinical psychology. The hypothesis that people have a very general view of others is contained in the work of Freud and other clinicians. Their view is that a person's basic interactions with his or her parents create a general view of what later interaction partners are like.

Consider the case of a person whose parents were very abusive, both verbally and physically. It would not be very surprising to learn that such a person as an adult is suspicious and not very trusting of others. In essence, this person tends to think that all others are abusive, as his or her parents were. Clinicians and self-help groups have theorized that children whose parents were alcoholics develop a particular view of others. These children as adults have a strong need to help and protect others; they also have difficulty with intimacy and closeness.

In a related vein, recent work on attachment style (Hazan & Shaver, 1987) emphasizes a similar theme. In this literature, interactions with a caregiver very early in life shape a person's expectancies later in life concerning others, particularly romantic partners.

Needed are data on how the parent treated the child and how the child (now an adult) sees others. The use of retrospective data from the adult child to measure prior parental behavior might contain the perceiver effect, and so it would be problematic. Thus, the measurement of parental treatment of the child should not be obtained from the child. From such a study, one could correlate parental treatment of the child with the perceiver effect of the child as an adult.

A more social-psychological notion is that the perceiver effect reflects the personality of one's close friends. That is, people tend to see others as they see their friends. According to this view, significant others serve to form a "floating average." The Kenny and Kashy (in press) study can be used to evaluate this hypothesis. We correlated the perceiver effect with how friends were seen by others. These correlations were very weak, and so this study does not provide much support for the "close friend as generalized other" hypothesis.

The Group Stereotype Interpretation

Assimilation reflects the view that "they are all alike." However, the perceiver effect may not be a generalized expectancy that a person has for *all* others; rather, it may be a local expectancy for the group that the person is rating. If the targets share some common bond (e.g., all are members of the same sorority or athletic team), there may be a tendency for the perceiver to see them as similar. The assimilation effect reflects the different stereotypes that perceivers have formed for different groups. The stereotype of a perceiver changes when a different group is being rated. In contrast, the generalized-other view is that the stereotype applies to all of humanity.

It should be noted that if all perceivers share the same stereotype, then the perceiver effect does not reflect a person's stereotype of the group; the stereotype is reflected only in the group mean. The perceiver effect reflects the stereotype that individuals have formed toward the group only when the stereotypes differ across individuals.

Consider the following example. Imagine that 20 college professors rate the photographs of 20 rock musicians on how intelligent they are. So professors are the perceivers and musicians are the targets. If all of the professors are equally prejudiced against the musicians, this prejudice should reveal itself in a low mean rating that professors give to musicians. However, if there are differences in the level of prejudice among the professors, these differences in stereotypes should reveal themselves in differences in the perceiver effect. Those with low perceiver effects (i.e., those who see musicians as low in intelligence) should be more prejudiced against musicians. So if there are differences in the level of prejudice, the perceiver effect would reflect the person's stereotype about the group. Better put, a person's perceiver effect reflects how his or her stereotype differs from other people's stereotypes.

If the measure is affective (e.g., how much the perceiver likes the target), then the perceiver effect reflects how much the person likes those who are in the group. Because "cohesiveness" can be defined as an individual's attraction to the group, the perceiver effect can be viewed as an individual-difference measure of cohesiveness.

Evidence Supporting the Group Stereotype View

There is strong evidence that a person's perceiver effect changes when different targets are being rated. Campbell, Miller, Lubetsky, and O'Connell (1964) examined the correlation of the perceiver effect in the ratings of college acquaintances with the perceiver effect in the ratings of strangers' photographs. They found that the correlations tended to be very small and usually not significantly different from zero. Thus, their study provides convincing evidence that the perceiver effect is not global, but changes according to the type of target.

A second piece of evidence is the over-time correlation of the perceiver effect. If the stereotype reflects the general perception of others, then the stability should be very large. But if the stereotype is more local, then the stereotype of the group may change over time as the individual begins to see the group in different ways. Presumably, even if the local stereotype were to change, most of the change would occur early.

Two studies can be used to investigate the stability of the perceiver effect. In one (Kenny et al., 1992, Study 2), people rated each other before interacting and after a one-on-one interaction. For those factors in which the perceiver accounted for at least 10% of the total variance, the average correlation of the perceiver effect over time was .64. These ratings took place within an hour. So there is evidence for changes in the perceiver effect. Montgomery (1984) examined students' ratings of leadership at three points during the semester. The perceiver–perceiver correlation between the first two times was .51, and the correlation between the last two times was .81. So this study likewise shows changes in the perceiver effect, but it also demonstrates that eventually the perceiver effect stabilizes.

The results from these two studies, as well as the results from Campbell et al. (1964), do provide strong evidence for the group stereotype notion of the perceiver effect. If the generalized-other view of the perceiver effect were true, then the correlations should have been near 1. Perhaps initially people apply a general stereotype to targets, and over time they acquire a particular stereotype for the group.

Ingroup and Outgroup Perceptions

Recently, social psychologists have given extensive attention to the question of ingroup–outgroup perception. To return to the example of college professors and rock musicians, if a professor is perceiving another professor or if a musician is perceiving another musician, these perceptions are "ingroup" perceptions. But if a person perceives a member of the other group (a professor is perceiving a musician or a musician is perceiving a professor), the perception is an "outgroup" perception. If the perceiver effect reflects the group stereotype, there should be a negative correlation between the perceiver effect for ingroup targets and the perceiver effect for outgroup targets: A fair judge should give equal ratings to ingroup and outgroup members, whereas a prejudiced judge should evaluate ingroup members favorably and outgroup members unfavorably.

The most systematic attempt to look for such a negative correlation was a study conducted by Kashy (1988). In a laboratory study, she created a four-person Red team and a four-person Green team, and these two teams competed in a trivia game. After the game was completed, subjects rated one another. Kashy obtained the usual ingroup favorability result: People evaluated ingroup members more favorably than they did outgroup members. However, the correlation in perceiver effects across groups was very positive, approaching 1.00. There was no evidence for the predicted negative correlation. Similar failures to find negative correlations were also obtained in more naturalistic studies of ingroup–outgroup perceptions (Whitley, Schofield, & Snyder, 1984; Yzerbyt, 1988).

There are two explanations for the failure to find the predicted negative correlation. To obtain the negative correlation between the perceiver effect for ingroup and outgroup members, there must be differential endorsement of the stereotype. If all members endorse the stereotype equally, then the correlation is not negative. Second, it seems likely (as noted earlier) that about 50% of the variance in perceiver effects can be accounted for by response set. If the same response set component is in both ingroup and outgroup ratings, the lowest that the ingroup–outgroup perceiver correlation would be is zero, and not -1.00.

The ideal study would be one in which there is differential endorsement of the stereotype and this endorsement of the stereotype is independently measured. The stereotype can then be correlated with the difference between ingroup and outgroup perceiver effects.

In sum, despite the disappointing results from the ingroup–outgroup area, the bulk of the evidence supports the group stereotype explanation of the perceiver effect. The perceiver effect reflects the perceiver's stereotype of the particular group being rated.

Conclusion

There is the troubling worry that perceiver variance does not reflect how the perceiver sees others, but rather how the perceiver assigns numbers to people. Some perceivers may be more inclined to use large numbers and others small numbers. The problem of response set in the perceiver effect is reintroduced when reciprocity is discussed in Chapter 6, and when assumed similarity is discussed in Chapter 9.

Classically, assimilation has been viewed as a directional phenomenon. If two targets, Z and H, are assimilated, one is the anchor and the other the object of assimilation. So the perception of Z is moved closer to the perception of the anchor, H. In this chapter, the perceiver effect represents a target that may be real, like the self or a significant other, or imagined, like the generalized other or a stereotype. It is this real or imagined other that serves as the anchor in the assimilation process.

It appears that assimilation effects are more than artifacts that can be attributed to response set. The research evidence supports the view that the perceiver effect reflects an expectation or stereotype of what others are like. Supportive of this hypothesis is that assimilation effects appear to decline over time.

There are two different approaches to the perceiver effect. First, it may reflect what others are typically like—the generalized other. The generalized other may reflect the self, or it may reflect an amalgam of perceptions of significant others in the person's life. Alternatively, assimilation effects may be less global and more local. They may be reflecting how one views a particular group. The evidence is more supportive of the group stereotype model.

The perceiver effect, which has received very limited study, deserves a more concentrated focus. Consider two recent and related examples. The health psychologist John Barefoot (1991) has theorized that the perceiver effect in the perception of hostility may lead to greater risk of heart disease. Research has shown that people who act in a very hostile fashion are more susceptible to heart disease. Barefoot believes that differences in hostility can be attributed to expectations that people have. That is, some people expect that others are going to treat them hostilely, and this expectation then creates its own reality. The expectation of hostility is nothing more than the perceiver effect of hostility. So the perceiver effect may well correlate with how people die!

In related work, Dodge and Coie (1987) have shown that adolescent boys who are labeled as aggressive by their peers are more likely to label the behaviors of others as aggressive. Thus, these boys have a perceiver effect, and they overestimate the aggressive intent of their peers. Thus, part of the reason for adolescent antisocial behavior is the perceiver effect. This example and the preceding one demonstrate that the perceiver effect has important life consequences for people.

Notes

1. Sometimes perceivers assume that the targets are very different from one another. In this case, perceivers are said to *contrast* the targets. Contrast effects are not generally found in rating data, but if they did exist they would be indicated by *negative* variance in perceiver effects.

2. Because the correlation is between two measures of the same construct and so can be viewed as a reliability coefficient, there is no need to square the correlation to determine how much variance is explained. The variance explained is simply the correlation.

3. Another possible source of response set is an anchoring-effect hypothesis. When subjects use a response scale, they place the first target rated near the midpoint of the scale. So if subjects rate targets in a different order, that creates a pseudo-perceiver effect. Such a hypothesis can be tested by correlating a person's perceiver effect with the target effect of the first target rated by the person. If the correlation is negative, there is support for the anchoring-effect interpretation of the perceiver effect.

4. Guilford (1954) also recommended placing all the positive traits on the left side of the page.

5. In both the Zaccaro et al. (1991) and the Chapdelaine et al. (in press) studies, some evidence suggested that the target variance (relative to the relationship variance) may be enhanced by using ranks. Rankings may enhance consensus, whereas ratings may enhance uniqueness. That is, rankings may distort the relationship effect in ratings.

6. I am grateful to Patrick Sullivan, who first made this suggestion to me.

Chapter 4

CONSENSUS

A fundamental topic in social science is the extent to which two observers or perceivers agree with each other in their impressions of a common target. Imagine two people, Mary and Susan, who are asked to judge on a 9-point scale how friendly Helen is. At issue is the extent to which Mary's rating of Helen agrees with Susan's rating of Helen or, using the notation developed in Chapter 1, $M(H) = S(H)$. This question is often called "agreement," but because people can agree about nonsocial objects, the term "consensus" is preferable. ("Consensus" has a different but related meaning in attribution theory that is not intended in this book.)

Quite clearly, the consensus question is closely related to the accuracy question. It should, however, be realized that consensus does not necessarily imply accuracy. A father and a mother can agree that their newborn child will win a Nobel Prize, but the child is not likely to win that prize. Generally, however, accuracy implies consensus. At the limit, this must be the case; that is, if two people are both exactly accurate, they must be in consensus. In social perception, exact accuracy is rare, and only partial accuracy is the norm (Kenny & Albright, 1987). It is both theoretically (Hastie & Rasinski, 1988) and empirically (Kenrick & Stringfield, 1980) possible for two perceivers not to agree, with both being partially accurate. If there are two different factors that determine behavior to which the two perceivers have differential access, they can disagree, yet both can be partially accurate. So, technically, consensus is neither a necessary nor a sufficient condition for accuracy.

Some presentations of consensus mix "self–peer" agreement (agreement between a person's view of a target and that target's view of him-

Parts of this chapter are adapted from Kenny (1991) and Kenny, Albright, Malloy, and Kashy (in press). Copyrights 1991 and 1994 by the American Psychological Association. Adapted by permission.

self or herself) with "peer–peer" agreement (agreement between two people about a third person). Although there are great similarities in the two sets of relationships, there are theoretical and empirical reasons (John & Robins, 1993) to expect differences. Thus, in this chapter, only peer–peer agreement is considered. Self–peer or self–other agreement is discussed in Chapter 9.

This chapter is divided into five sections. In the first, I provide a historical review of consensus studies. In the second, I consider the measurement of consensus. In the third, I review the results from 32 studies of consensus. In the fourth, I present a conceptual model of person perception that explains the different sources of consensus (Kenny, 1991). Finally, in the fifth section, I attempt to explain the results from the empirical review using the conceptual model. The major focus in the empirical review is the relationship between consensus and acquaintance.

Historical Review

Historically, there are four interwoven traditions that have studied consensus: research in social psychology, personality, observer ratings, and informant accuracy. These four research areas are briefly reviewed.

Social Psychology

Within social psychology, there has been considerable interest in the extent to which person perception is driven by the stimulus or driven by the perceiver's internal processes. This question has been described in various ways. For instance, researchers following Dornbusch, Hastorf, Richardson, Muzzy, and Vreeland (1965) have referred to the "eye of the beholder"; that is, perception reflects the beliefs and expectations of the perceiver, and not the characteristics of the target. Higgins and Bargh (1987) have discussed the issue of whether social perception is data-driven or theory-driven. Research in the area of consensus has been very important in this debate.

The most influential study in this area is that by Dornbusch et al. (1965). They studied an unspecified number of 9- to 11-year-old male residents of a summer camp, who had known each other for only 2 to 3 weeks. Each child was asked to describe in words the other camp residents, and the responses were coded into 69 categories. Dornbusch et al. (1965) found very little consensus and concluded that "the most powerful influence on interpersonal description is the manner in which the perceiver structures his interpersonal world" (p. 440).

The Dornbusch et al. (1965) study was followed up by Bourne (1977) and Park (1986). Bourne, using only 17 people, replicated the Dornbusch et al. study. Instead of using relatively unacquainted children, he used well-acquainted adults, and he used rating scales as well as free descriptions. Like Dornbusch et al., Bourne found low levels of consensus. Park (1986) examined consensus in a more controlled environment than previous studies had employed, and found higher levels of consensus than the earlier studies.

Motivational factors seem to influence consensus. Work by Touhey (1972) and Rozelle and Baxter (1981) showed that experimental instructions to increase the subject's motivation to be accurate also increased consensus.

Personality

Researchers in personality have relied primarily on self-report inventories to measure individual differences. However, as reviewed by Wiggins (1973), some researchers (e.g., Cattell) have supplemented self-report measures with peer ratings, and others (e.g., Norman) have primarily relied on peer-rating inventories.

Over the last decade or so, there has been a virtual explosion of personality studies employing peer ratings (Kenrick & Funder, 1988). To a large extent, these studies have been undertaken in response to the attack on personality. For instance, Bourne (1977) claimed to show that there is little consensus and thus that personality does not exist. Subsequently, numerous personality researchers (Funder, 1987; Kenrick & Funder, 1988; Kenrick & Stringfield, 1980; Moskowitz & Schwarz, 1982) have argued that consensus exists in personality judgments and that it demonstrates an empirical basis for individual differences.

Observer Ratings

Social scientists have long used observers to rate or code social behavior. As biologists use mass spectrometers and chemists use electron microscopes, the most valued "instrument" used by social scientists is the human observer.

Initially, classical test theory was applied to human observers, who were treated as if they were items on a test. It became clear that human observers were subject to leniency and halo biases that were less problematic with nonhuman methods. Models of the rating process were proposed by Guilford (1954) and Stanley (1961), and were in large part subsumed by Cronbach, Gleser, Nanda, and Rajaratnam's (1972) generalizability theory.

A second tradition besides classical test theory is the multitrait–multimethod matrix (Campbell & Fiske, 1959), in which the perceiver is treated as a method of measurement. Consensus between a pair of perceivers is called "convergent validation" within this tradition.

Researchers in areas other than personality have used peer ratings as a basic measure. Developmental psychologists interested in popularity, social skills, and social withdrawal have used peer ratings. Also, in industrial psychology, performance appraisal often involves having more than one person evaluate a given target.

Informant Accuracy

Recently, anthropologists have become quite interested in consensus. In their research, they repeatedly ask informants how they feel about various issues. The assumption is made that when these local informants all give the same answer, there must exist a culture to which the informants belong. Romney, Weller, and Batchelder (1986) have proposed that consensus can be used to identify culture.

In related work, Campbell (1961, 1979) has proposed that what creates a scientific culture is consensus. Interestingly, Campbell has compared scientists to tribe members and scientific leaders to chiefs.

The Measurement of Consensus

In the literature, there are three different approaches to the measurement of consensus: discrepancy, correlation, and variance approaches. Each is considered below.

Discrepancy

By far the simplest measure of consensus (but, ironically, the most difficult to interpret) is the discrepancy score. A discrepancy score measures the extent to which two perceivers disagree in their ratings of a common target. So if John thinks that Mary is friendly and Peter does not, there is a discrepancy. For a dichotomous variable, discrepancy is the inverse of agreement, and so the two measures are interchangeable: Discrepancy implies a total lack of agreement. For a continuous variable, a discrepancy score does not indicate a total lack of agreement, but rather some level of disagreement.

A discrepancy measure can be defined as the *absolute* difference between the ratings by two perceivers of the same target. A discrepancy score can be computed across targets by summing across them. Alternatively, the discrepancies can be squared, then summed, and finally square-rooted to obtain a distance measure.

One difficulty with the discrepancy measure is that there is no natural baseline to enable investigators to determine whether the level of consensus is above chance levels. Dornbusch et al. (1965) developed a creative baseline measure: They asked whether two perceivers agreed in their descriptions of the same target as often as two perceivers agreed in their descriptions of two different targets. The former measure is called "2-on-1" agreement, and the latter "2-on-2" agreement. They also proposed a "1-on-2" agreement measure: To what extent does the perceiver agree with himself or herself in rating two targets? Thus, 1-on-2 agreement measures the extent to which a perceiver assimilates targets. The appropriate baseline for 2-on-1 agreement is 2-on-2. The 2-on-1 versus 2-on-2 comparison assesses the extent to which perceivers agree at more than chance levels. The Dornbusch et al. 2-on-2 baseline has been used by Touhey (1972), Bourne (1977), Rozelle and Baxter (1981), and Park (1986).

The primary problem with discrepancy scores is that they are influenced by response set. Because Cronbach (1955; Kenny & Albright, 1987) has made this argument, it is only briefly restated here. Imagine two perceivers (*A* and *B*) who rate six targets (*C* through *H*) on an 8-point scale. Person *A*'s ratings of *C* through *H* are 3, 5, 6, 4, 3, and 4, respectively; *B*'s ratings are 6, 8, 9, 7, 6, and 7, respectively. The average discrepancy score between perceivers *A* and *B* is 3.0. For the 2-on-2 Dornbusch et al. measure, the average discrepancy score is slightly lower, 2.8. The 2-on-1 discrepancy is larger than the 2 on 2, and so the two perceivers appear to agree less than would be expected by chance. However, it can be seen that perceiver *A*'s ratings are always 3 points lower than *B*'s. Once this adjustment is made, there is exact agreement. Because the mean level of a perceiver's ratings is often of little psychological interest, and because the discrepancy score is very sensitive to the mean difference between perceivers, the discrepancy measure of consensus can be very misleading.

Correlation

When a group of targets is rated by two or more perceivers, a correlation can be used to index consensus. The correlational measure of consensus has the advantage of a natural baseline of zero, and because the perceivers' means are subtracted, response set does not affect it. Also, the interpretation of a correlation coefficient is relatively straightforward: A correlation of 1 indicates exact relative agreement, and a correlation of 0 indicates no agreement beyond chance levels.

The correlational measure of consensus is used commonly by personality psychologists. An example of a study that used a correlational measure of consensus is that by Woodruffe (1984), who had 66 members of a class recruit 10 close acquaintances, each of whom rated the member who chose him or her. Thus, for each of the 66 class members there were 10 ratings, one from each acquaintance. The class members were the targets, and the acquaintances were the perceivers. Evidently, Woodruffe arbitrarily labeled the friends as perceivers 1 through 10 and then intercorrelated the ratings with 10 variables, resulting in 45 correlations. The average of these correlations was used to measure consensus, and its value was .22.

Although a correlational measure is greatly superior to a discrepancy measure of consensus, it nonetheless has drawbacks. For example, note that for each target, Woodruffe (1984) arbitrarily assigned perceivers to the positions 1 through 10. Any different assignment pattern would probably yield a different average between-perceiver correlation. An intraclass correlation, not an ordinary correlation, would have been more appropriate for this study.

Variance

The variance measure gives the amount of variation in the ratings that is determined by the target. For each target, the mean rating, averaged across perceivers, is computed. If these means differ from target to target (i.e., if they vary), there is evidence of consensus. Perhaps the first use of a variance measure was in the Norman and Goldberg (1966) study. These researchers had perceivers rank-order the targets. They then computed the variance in the means for targets and subtracted what the variance would have been if the perceivers had assigned ranks randomly.

Generalizability theory (Cronbach et al., 1972) can be used to develop a variance measure of consensus. Consider the case in which there are n perceivers and m different targets. To determine the variance that can be attributed to target, a two-way analysis of variance is computed in which the two factors are perceiver and target. From this analysis, one can compute the proportion of variance that is attributable to target by dividing the estimated target variance by the sum of the estimated perceiver variance, target variance, and perceiver × target variance. The ratio of target variance to total variance can be interpreted as a correlation: If one were to sample perceivers and targets randomly, the proportion of target variance would represent the correlation between two perceivers.

Much of the research on social perception has employed a reciprocal design in which each person serves as both a perceiver and a target, whereas in the classical design a set of perceivers rates a set of targets, and the perceivers and the targets are different people (Kenny & Albright, 1987). When a reciprocal design is undertaken, complications arise in the computation of the variance components. First, there are missing data because people do not rate themselves; even if they do, those data should be set aside, because self-ratings may be qualitatively different from other ratings. Second, there is nonindependence in the data (Kenny & Judd, 1986), because the level at which John rates Joe may well be correlated with the level at which Joe rates John. My colleagues and I have developed procedures for estimating the variance components for reciprocal designs (Kenny, 1981, 1988; Warner, Kenny, & Stoto, 1979), and these have been included in the Social Relations Model (SRM). Actually, SRM can be viewed as the application of generalizability theory to data gathered from reciprocal designs (Malloy & Kenny, 1986). A detailed description of the estimation of the variance components is presented in Appendix B.

A variance measure is somewhat less interpretable than a correlational measure. Fortunately, a variance can be converted into a correlation. For instance, the target variance divided by the total variance estimates the correlation for a design in which each target is judged by a different pair of perceivers.

A major disadvantage of the variance measure is that computational difficulties often require specialized computer software. There is also the possibility of anomalous values. Estimates of variance components can be negative, but negative variance estimates usually indicate small or no population variances. The advantages of a variability measure are that it generalizes across targets and perceivers and has a baseline of zero. Moreover, the proportion of variance that is attributable to target can be viewed as a correlation.

In this chapter, the proportion of variance that can be attributed to target is used as the measure of consensus. Such a statistic can be interpreted as the average correlation in ratings between two perceivers, given that each target is rated by a different pair of perceivers. It represents the percentage of the variance in an individual's rating that can be attributed to the target.

Empirical Review

My colleagues and I (Kenny, Albright, Malloy, & Kashy, in press) conducted the most comprehensive survey of consensus to date. This section presents the results from our summary. We examined the level of consensus from 32 studies with 2934 subjects using 407 traits. Thirteen of the studies examined consensus over time. In each of these over-time studies, the results refer to the same set of people across time, and so any people who missed one or more times were eliminated.[1]

To qualify for inclusion, a study had to meet several criteria. First, each perceiver had to evaluate multiple targets, and each target had to be judged by multiple perceivers. Twenty-three of the studies employed round-robin designs (see Chapter 2, Table 2.5a); in such a design, each person judges everyone in the group. Other designs were also used (Kenny, 1990), and six of the remaining nine studies employed block designs (see Table 2.5b). In a block design, the people are divided into two groups, and each person in one group rates all those who are in the other group. The second criterion for inclusion in this review was that for each study, the proportion of target variance had to be measured. A list of the 32 studies is presented in Table 4.1, and a brief description of each is given in Appendix A.

As throughout this text, the Big Five factor classification is used. Factor I is called Extroversion, Factor II is called Agreeableness, Factor III is called Conscientiousness, Factor IV is called Emotional Stability, and Factor V is called Culture.

Besides trait type, a second variable considered in the summary of studies was the level of acquaintance between the perceiver and the target. Three different levels of acquaintance, as initially discussed in Chapter 1, were used. The first level is zero acquaintance (Albright et al., 1988), in which the perceiver and target have no prior interaction history. The second level of acquaintance is short-term acquaintance, in which the perceiver and target meet and interact for a brief time (usually no more than an hour). Either these interactions can be one-on-one with no one else present, or they can take place in a group. This category includes studies of classroom groups even if they met throughout the semester. The final level of acquaintance is long-term acquaintance, in which most of the people have known each other for years. A typical study of this type would involve a group of people living in a college sorority or fraternity.

Using this classification system, we (Kenny et al., in press) could classify each of the 32 studies into the different levels of acquaintance. In 13 of the studies, the perceivers rated the targets at more than one

TABLE 4.1. List of 32 Studies in Empirical Review

Albright (1990)	Kenny & DePaulo (1990), applicant
Albright, Kenny, & Malloy (1988), Study 1	Kenny & DePaulo (1990), interviewer
Albright, Kenny, & Malloy (1988), Study 2	Kenny, Horner, Kashy, & Chu (1992), Study 1
Albright, Kenny, & Malloy (1988), Study 3	Kenny, Horner, Kashy, & Chu (1992), Study 2
Albright-Malloy (1988)	Kenny, Horner, Kashy, & Chu (1992), Study 3
Anderson (1985)	Latané (1987)
Campbell, Miller, Lubetsky, & O'Connell (1964)	Levesque (1990)
Dantchik (1985)	Malloy (1987a)
DePaulo, Kenny, Hoover, Webb, & Oliver (1987)	Malloy & Albright (1990)
DiPilato (1990)	McGillan (1980)
Hallmark (1991)	Montgomery (1984)
Hallmark & Kenny (1989)	Oliver (1989)
Kashy (1988)	Park & Judd (1989)
Kenny (1992)	Reno & Kenny (1992)
Kenny & Bernstein (1982)	Rothbart & Singer (1988)
	Schill & Thomsen (1987)
	Yingling (1989)

Note. For details on these studies, see Appendix A. Adapted from Kenny, Albright, Malloy, and Kashy (in press). Copyright 1994 by the American Psychological Association. Adapted by permission.

time, and these studies are called the "longitudinal" studies. Four of these studies were in two different classifications of acquaintance (generally zero and short-term group). Also, it is unclear what the proper classification of wave 1 of the Albright-Malloy (1988) study is (it being a mixture of zero and short-term group acquaintance); thus wave 1 from that study is not included in the cross-sectional review, but is included in the longitudinal review. The review of the studies is divided into two sections: one for the cross-sectional results, and one for the longitudinal results.

Cross-Sectional Results

The review of the cross-sectional results is divided into four sections, covering studies of zero acquaintance; short-term acquaintance, one-on-one interactions; short-term acquaintance, group interactions; and long-term acquaintance. For each study, the results of the variance partitioning are presented for the Big Five factors.

To determine consensus for each of the five factors, the mean consensus across traits was computed for each study, and medians across studies were computed. Table 4.2 presents the levels of consensus for the Big Five factors by the four levels of acquaintance.

Zero Acquaintance

Table 4.2 presents the results of nine zero-acquaintance studies. In seven of the nine studies, the targets were physically present in the room with the perceiver; in one study, the targets were on videotape (Kenny, Horner, Kashy, & Chu, 1992, Study 1); and in one study, the targets were photographed (Latané, 1987).

The results for Factor I, Extroversion, show relatively high levels of consensus; nearly 30% of the variance in ratings of Extroversion is target-based. The factor with the next highest level of consensus is Conscientiousness, but its size is only half that of Extroversion. The factors of Emotional Stability and Culture show low levels of consensus, and the factor of Agreeableness shows hardly any consensus at all.

Short-Term Acquaintance, One-on-One Interactions

Across nine studies of short-term acquaintance, one-on-one interactions, the level of consensus for the factors is rather low. Averaging across the five factors, the level of consensus is only .070, and the highest level of consensus is only .083 for Extroversion. One-on-one interactions with strangers produce relatively low levels of consensus.

In one-on-one interactions, the level of consensus is considerably lower for Extroversion and Conscientiousness than it is for those factors in the zero-acquaintance studies. So gathering more data about

TABLE 4.2. Median Consensus Estimates (Proportions of Target Variance) for the Big Five Factors in the Cross-Sectional Studies

	n^a	N^b	I	II	III	IV	V
Zero acquaintance	9	798	.273	.032	.134	.085	.070
Short-term acquaintance							
One-on-one	9	644	.083	.082	.034	.070	.079
Group	13	1250	.320	.096	.156	.104	.141
Long-term acquaintance	5	645	.286	.270	.265	.263	.290

Note. Factor numbers: I, Extroversion; II, Agreeableness; III, Conscientiousness; IV, Emotional Stability; V, Culture. Adapted from Kenny et al. (in press). Copyright 1994 by the American Psychological Association. Adapted by permission.
[a]The number of studies.
[b]The number of perceivers.

a target appears to lower consensus for those two factors. Compared with the zero-acquaintance studies, there is virtually no change in consensus for Emotional Stability or Culture, but Agreeableness does show an increase. If the source of consensus at zero acquaintance is a set of stereotypes, then the perception of targets in one-on-one interactions is not based on stereotypes to the same extent as it is in zero acquaintance. Perception is more individuated, but evidently target behaviors are not very consistent across interaction partners.

Short-Term Acquaintance, Group

In 13 short-term acquaintance studies, people interacted in groups. Extroversion shows the greatest level of consensus. Conscientiousness is a distant second, and close behind is Culture. Agreeableness and Emotional Stability both have consensus levels of about .10. The pattern of results for these studies mirrors that for the zero-acquaintance studies, but consensus is somewhat higher in the short-term group studies.

The similarity between the short-term group and zero-acquaintance results is not that surprising, because a short-term group study is not very different from a zero-acquaintance study. Participation may be the only cue added in many group studies. Dabbs and Ruback (1987) have shown that when individuals participate more equally in groups, there is less consensus in ratings. Because Extroversion information is picked up with minimal interaction, group interaction may add relatively little information to perceivers' impressions of targets.

In some studies, the situation was designed to provide particular information to the perceivers about the targets' standing on a trait. For instance, in both the DiPilato (1990) and Kashy (1988) studies, the subjects engaged in intellectual tasks. In both studies, there are relatively high levels of consensus on Culture (.30). So, unless the situation provides a context to elicit information concerning a specific factor, the profile of consensus from a short-term group study is likely to resemble closely the profile from a zero-acquaintance study.

Long-Term Acquaintance

Only five studies examined consensus among people who had known each other for an extended time. However, these studies had large sample sizes, involving a total of 645 people.

The level of consensus from these studies is quite homogeneous, averaging to .275. We (Kenny et al., in press) found, as did Paunonen (1989), that among well-acquainted individuals there is little difference across the traits in the level of consensus. Interestingly, for Extroversion the level of consensus is only slightly higher than it is at zero acquaintance, and less than the level of consensus in short-term groups. Increasing acquaintance does not appear to increase consensus for Extroversion.

Summary of Cross-Sectional Results

Several general trends appear in Table 4.2. First, when there are differences in the factors for a given level of acquaintance, there is more consensus in the ratings of Extroversion than in those for any other factor. This is particularly true for zero-acquaintance and short-term group interactions. Second, and counterintuitively, social interaction does not always result in an increase in consensus, but can actually result in a decrease. This can be seen by comparing the short-term one-on-one results to the zero-acquaintance results. Third, short-term group interactions result in greater levels of consensus than short-term one-on-one interactions for all five factors. The most likely explanation is that there is greater overlap in stimulus information in group than in one-on-one interactions. In group studies perceivers are exposed to the same information, whereas in one-on-one studies perceivers are probably exposed to different information. Fourth, long-term acquaintance results in uniform but modest levels of consensus. Except for Extroversion, consensus is greatest with long-term acquaintance. The interpretation of the cross-sectional results is discussed in more detail later in this chapter.

Longitudinal Results

Now considered are the results of 12 over-time studies that measured consensus. Note that the Kenny and DePaulo (1990) interviewer study is not considered here, because the level of consensus was so low (the mean being .01) that there was no room for any temporal trends.

Table 4.3 presents summary information about the patterns of change in these studies. For each factor, a linear trend (i.e., a measure of whether consensus increased or decreased) over time was computed. If the study included a zero-acquaintance condition, that wave was dropped because our purpose was to study the effect of acquaintance on consensus.

To interpret the results in Table 4.3, recall that even if there were no trends over time, the expectation would be that 50% of the studies would show an increase. As can be seen in Table 4.3, there is a

TABLE 4.3. Summary of the Longitudinal Results

Variable	% studies that show increase
Acquaintance level	
Laboratory studies	46
Classroom studies	71
Factor	
Extroversion	33
Agreeableness	50
Conscientiousness	56
Emotional Stability	56
Culture	62

Note. Adapted from Kenny et al. (in press). Copyright 1994 by the American Psychological Association. Adapted by permission.

tendency toward no increase in consensus over time in the laboratory studies, but there is a hint of an increase in consensus in classroom studies. (Because there was only one residential longitudinal study, it is not included in this part of the summary.) We (Kenny et al., in press) have offered the following interpretation of the results from the laboratory studies: The degree of acquaintance was minimal in these studies, and so very limited information was gained about the target. Moreover, these laboratory situations did not provide much information about a person's personality besides Extroversion, and that information was picked up very quickly. The classroom situation did allow for interaction over a longer time. Moreover, people were not as constrained by the situation as they were in the laboratory, and so they probably interacted more naturally. The classroom situation also allowed perceivers to gain information about Conscientiousness and Culture that could not be readily ascertained in the typical laboratory experiment. However, it should be noted that the level of acquaintance by the final waves may have been minimal even in these studies. For most of the classroom studies, people interacted for no more than 2 or 3 hours.

Table 4.3 also presents the results separately for the five factors. The pattern is fairly clear: Extroversion and Agreeableness show no increase over time, whereas the other three factors do show an increase. So extended interaction with targets may well lead to increased consensus for Conscientiousness, Emotional Stability, and Culture.

Although the results in Table 4.3 are suggestive, it should be realized that the longitudinal patterns are inconsistent (Kenny et al., in press). There is then little basis for concluding from these 12 longitudinal studies that increased acquaintance leads to an increase in consensus.

Before an attempt is made to interpret the longitudinal and cross-sectional results, a general model is presented. This model can be used as a framework to understand the puzzling findings that have been encountered in the empirical summary.

A General Model of Consensus: The Weighted-Average Model

In this section, a comprehensive mathematical formulation of the various factors that determine the level of consensus is presented. The model, called the "Weighted-Average Model" (WAM; Kenny, 1991), has been developed in an attempt to clarify the anomalies found in the empirical review. WAM can be used to predict the level of consensus as well as other aspects of interpersonal perception. It is also used in the discussion of uniqueness in Chapter 5, target accuracy in Chapter 7, and self–other agreement in Chapter 9. The technical details of WAM (including two additional parameters not discussed here) are presented in Appendix C.

It is important to differentiate WAM from SRM. WAM is a theoretical model that describes the processes by which trait impressions are formed. SRM is a statistical model that partitions variance into perceiver, target, and relationship.

Model Parameters

Before the formal model is presented, the nine factors that combine to determine consensus must be defined. Table 4.4 lists these parameters, and a brief description of each is presented below.

- "Acquaintance," or n. Acquaintance is the sheer amount of information (i.e., number of behavioral acts) to which the perceiver is exposed. Presumably, the more behaviors observed, the more perceivers should agree. Acquaintance is viewed as a quantitative variable.
- "Overlap," or q. To what extent do two perceivers observe the target simultaneously? That is, to what extent do the perceivers observe the same set of target behaviors? The overlap factor, which has been largely ignored, plays a pivotal role in determining the degree of consensus.

TABLE 4.4. Parameters of WAM

Parameter	Definition
n	Acquaintance (number of behavioral acts)
q	Overlap
r_1	Consistency
r_2	Similar meaning systems
w	Weight of physical-appearance stereotypes
r_3	Agreement about stereotypes
r_4	"Kernel of truth" in stereotypes
k	Weight of unique impression (extraneous information)
a	Communication

Note. In Kenny (1991), w was set to 0, and r_3 and r_4 were not present. Appendix C presents a fuller version of the model, in which r_3 and r_4 as defined here are labeled differently (see Table C.1).

- "Consistency," or r_1. How consistent is the target's behavior? If the target is friendly in one situation, would the target be friendly in another situation? Historically, personality researchers have taken consensus to be a measure of the extent to which the target's behavior is consistent, but it is shown below that consensus can exist even when the target's behaviors are inconsistent.
- "Similar meaning systems," or r_2. To what extent is an act given the same meaning by two perceivers? That is, if two perceivers see a target engage in a behavior, to what extent do they label that behavior in the same way?
- "Physical-appearance stereotypes," or w. To what extent do stereotypes about physical appearance (e.g., age, sex, ethnicity, vocal quality, physical attractiveness) influence impressions? It is well established that first impressions are affected by such stereotypes.
- "Agreement about stereotypes," or r_3. To what extent do the perceivers agree with each other in their stereotypes about physical appearance? Presumably, stereotypes are largely culturally driven, and there is likely to be high levels of agreement.
- "Validity of stereotypes," or r_4. To what extent do the stereotypes about physical appearance predict the behavior of the target being rated? In other words, is there a "kernel of truth" in those stereotypes?
- "Unique impression," or k. To what extent does the perceiver rate the target based on extraneous information, that is, information not based on the target's acts or appearance?
- "Communication," or a. To what extent do the perceivers share

with each other their impressions of the target? The ratings of two perceivers can be similar because they communicate their impressions to each other.

It is possible to relate all nine of these factors in a single mathematical model. A modified version of Anderson's (1981) weighted-average model is used; hence the name of the present model, "Weighted-Average Model." First, a brief review of Anderson's weighted-average model is presented. Imagine that a perceiver knows three facts about a target: She is a librarian, she is politically conservative, and she likes to dance. The perceiver is asked to rate how extroverted the target is. According to Anderson's weighted-average model, each fact has a scale value. The scale value, symbolized by s, states the impression that the perceiver would have of the target if there were no other information. Presumably for Extroversion, "being a librarian" would have a negative scale value, whereas "liking to dance" would have a positive scale value.

Also associated with each piece of information is a weight. The weights multiply the scale values and represent the importance or salience of the information. Anderson's weighted-average model states that the impression that a perceiver has of the target equals the sum of each scale value multiplied by a weight, and this sum is divided by the sum of the weights. This weighted-average model is now applied, in the form of WAM, to the measurement of consensus.

WAM assumes that a target engages in a series of behavioral acts (which include both verbal and nonverbal behaviors). The acts are designated as A's, and the target's physical appearance as P. A perceiver, who observes a subset of the A's and the target's P, is asked to judge that target on a given trait. Each act and the physical-appearance information is given a meaning, or in terms of Anderson's (1981) model, a scale value.

Two perceivers may attach different scale values to the same act and the same physical appearance. For instance, if they observe the same act (e.g., Dave losing his keys), one may infer that the act was dispositionally caused (Dave is forgetful), whereas the other may infer that the act was situationally caused (the keys fell out of Dave's pocket).

The perceiver's impression of the target is also influenced by the "unique impression," which represents that part of the perceiver's impression not caused by the target's acts or physical appearance. For instance, the perceiver may be favorably disposed toward the target because the perceiver is in a good mood that day or because the perceiver believes that all targets tend to have a high standing on the trait.

The unique impression in WAM is a broader concept than the "initial impression" in Anderson's (1981) formulation. In WAM, the unique impression represents all the information that a perceiver uses that is not based on the target's behavior. In Anderson's model, the initial impression represents a perceiver's impression of a target based on no information. The unique impression can change over time, whereas the initial impression cannot change.

The perceiver's impression of the target is assumed to be a weighted average of the scale values for the behaviors that the perceiver observes, the scale value of physical appearance, and the unique impression. It is assumed that each act is equally weighted. The equal-weighting assumption is made to simplify an already complex model. Ideally, future work with WAM will relax the equal-weighting assumption.

Figure 4.1 presents WAM in schematic form. There is one target who engages in three acts. Of course, real targets engage in many more acts in a few minutes, but for illustrative purposes only a few acts are chosen. The acts are labeled A_1 through A_3. Two perceivers observe a subset of the target's acts. The first perceiver views acts A_1 and A_2 and the second perceiver observes A_2 and A_3. Both perceivers view the target's physical appearance, P.

Each perceiver evaluates the target, and a meaning or a scale value s is attached to each act observed by each perceiver and to the target's physical appearance. Note that although both perceivers observe A_2, each attaches a different meaning to that act, and this is indicated by the

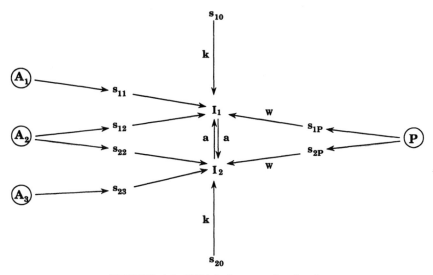

FIGURE 4.1. WAM. See text for details.

double subscripts. For example, s_{12} in Figure 4.1 is the scale value for A_2 as observed by perceiver 1. Each perceiver also attaches a different meaning, s_{1P} or s_{2P}, to the physical-appearance information, P. Also, each perceiver forms a unique impression of the target, denoted by s_{10} for perceiver 1 and s_{20} for perceiver 2. The scale values for the acts observed by the perceiver (equally weighted), the physical-appearance information, and the unique impression combine to form that perceiver's impression of a particular trait, I. The perceivers then communicate their impressions to each other, and they may thereby influence each other. This mutual influence is represented by the paths labeled a in Figure 4.1. The value of a can be negative; for instance, if the perceivers dislike each other, they might negatively influence one another.

The correlation between two perceivers' impressions across a set of targets is a function of the nine parameters described earlier and presented in Table 4.4. First is n, the number of acts that each perceiver observes, which is assumed to be the same for each perceiver. Second is q, the proportion of acts for the two perceivers that overlap. So if n is 40 and q is .75, then the two perceivers see nq, or 30, of the same acts. In Figure 4.1, q is .5 because each perceiver sees two acts, one of which (A_2) is the same. The third parameter is r_1, the degree to which a target's behavior is consistent. It measures the extent to which the same perceiver assigns similar scale values to two different acts. In Figure 4.1, it is the correlation between s_{11} and s_{12}. Fourth is r_2, the correlation between two perceivers' scale values for the same act. This parameter measures the similarity between the two perceivers' meaning systems. In Figure 4.1, it is the correlation between s_{12} and s_{22}.

There are three parameters that refer to the use of physical-appearance stereotypes. First is w, the weight attached to these stereotypes. Second is r_3, the degree to which perceivers agree in their stereotypes. In Figure 4.1, it is the correlation between s_{1P} and s_{2P}. Third is r_4, the degree to which the stereotype correlates with the perception of behavior. In Figure 4.1, it is the correlation between s_{1P} and s_{11}.

There are two final parameters in the model. First is k, the weight for the unique impression. Second is a, the degree to which the perceivers influence each other.

The equations that state the amount of consensus are presented in Appendix C. These equations express consensus, denoted as c, in terms of the nine parameters: acquaintance (n), overlap (q), consistency (r_1), similar meaning systems (r_2), weight given to stereotypes (w), similar stereotypes (r_3), validity of stereotypes (r_4), weight of the unique impression (k), and communication (a).[2] The equations are quite complex, but they have some important but nonobvious implications for the study of consensus. In the remainder of this section of the chapter, I explore these conclusions.

Implications of the Model

Before the implications of the model are considered, it is important to remember that the measure of consensus is the correlation between two perceivers' ratings across a set of targets. So if Zelda and Heidi rate 10 people whom they know in common, they would show consensus if their ratings of a trait across the 10 targets were correlated. In keeping with the focus of the chapter, the primary emphasis is on the relationship between consensus and acquaintance.

This section is quite difficult. Keeping track of nine parameters and what they each mean is not simple. To facilitate comprehension, the major conclusions of this section are printed in bold type.

Considered first are the implications of the model if it is assumed that perception is not determined by the unique impression or physical appearance, and that there is no communication between perceivers. Thus k, w, and a are set to zero, and the impression is entirely attributable to the perception of the target's behaviors.

If physical-appearance and unique-impression effects are absent, and if there is some consistency but less than perfect overlap, greater acquaintance leads to greater consensus. Consensus increases because of the increased reliability in the perceivers' impressions. That is, with increased acquaintance, a perceiver samples more of the target's acts and so forms a more reliable impression. This increase in sample size results in an increase in consensus only if there is some consistency in the target's behaviors and the two perceivers sample different target behaviors (i.e., overlap is less than perfect).

However, given high overlap, acquaintance does not always lead to increased consensus. The relationship between acquaintance and consensus as moderated by overlap is shown graphically in Figure 4.2. The following assumptions have been made: There is weak consistency ($r_1 = .05$) and moderately to very similar meaning systems ($r_2 = .5$). (These hypothetical values are consistent with the empirical work of Park, DeKay, & Kraus, 1994.) The relationship between acquaintance, or n, and consensus, or c, is presented for three values of the overlap parameter, or q. When there is perfect overlap ($q = 1$), consensus does not increase as acquaintance does. **When physical-appearance and unique-impression effects are absent, perfect overlap results in consensus being unrelated to acquaintance.** As overlap declines, acquaintance begins to have more of an effect on consensus.

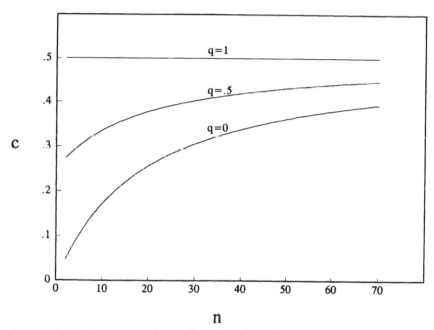

FIGURE 4.2. Consensus (c) as a function of overlap (q) and acquaintance (n).

The increase in consensus as a function of acquaintance can be attributed to the increased reliability because of the larger sample size of acts.

If both the unique-impression and physical-appearance information are added to the model, the relationship between acquaintance and consensus becomes much more complicated. At this stage, it is assumed that there is no "kernel of truth" ($r_4 = 0$), and that there is no communication ($a = 0$). As in Figure 4.2, the assumptions of weak consistency ($r_1 = .05$) and moderately to strongly similar meaning systems ($r_2 = .5$) have been made.

Still yet another correlation needs to be defined here. It is the degree of consensus between two perceivers when the target is judged without reference to the behavior of the target. That correlation, to be called r_5, can be shown to equal $r_3 w^2 / (w^2 + k^2)$. Basically, r_5 captures the degree to which stereotypes about physical appearance determine the perceivers' impression and the degree to which those stereotypes are shared.

Considered first is the case[3] in which $r_5 = r_2 = .5$. In this case, the nonbehavioral information is shared to the same degree as the behavioral information. As shown in Figure 4.3, when there is perfect overlap, there is no relationship between acquaintance and consensus: The function is perfectly flat, as it is in Figure 4.2 when there is

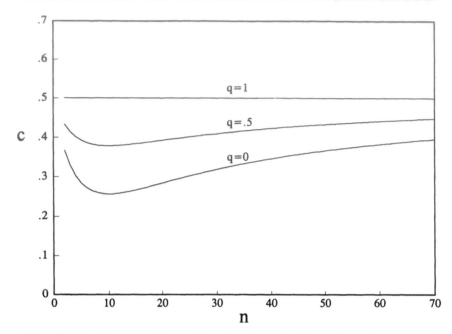

FIGURE 4.3. Consensus (c) as a function of overlap (q), moderately consensual stereotypes ($r_5 = r_2$), and acquaintance (n).

perfect overlap. As overlap declines, the function becomes increasingly concave or bent: Consensus first declines and then later increases. The decline is caused by the fact that physical-appearance information, which is shared, is given increasingly less weight. The increase is a result of the augmented reliability because of sample size. The degree of concavity in the function (i.e., the degree to which it is shaped like a bowl) depends on overlap: The less overlap, the greater the bend in the function.

If physical-appearance information is not given much weight or it is not very consensual ($r_5 < r_2$), then the relationship between consensus and acquaintance becomes stronger, as in Figure 4.4. As seen for all three values of the overlap parameter, the level of consensus increases as acquaintance increases. However, the increase is smaller when there is less overlap. **High overlap dampens the relationship between acquaintance and consensus.**

However, if physical-appearance information is given great weight and is highly consensual ($r_5 > r_2$), the relationship becomes increasingly concave, as in Figure 4.5. With very low acquaintance ($1 < n < 35$), there is even a negative relationship between acquaintance and consensus, but for more established relationships and low

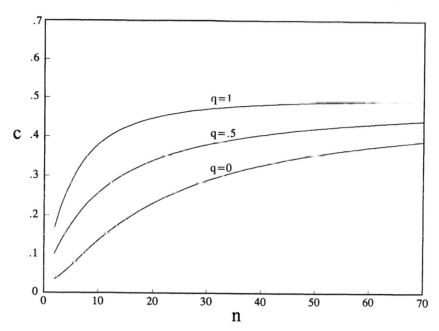

FIGURE 4.4. Consensus (c) as a function of overlap (q), weakly consensual stereotypes ($r_s < r_2$), and acquaintance (n).

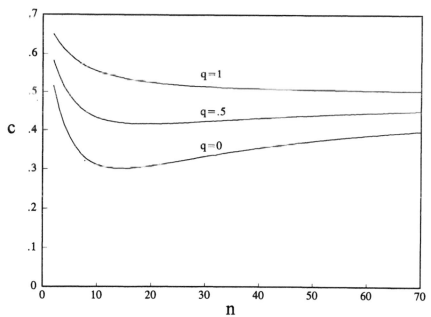

FIGURE 4.5. Consensus (c) as a function of overlap (q), strongly consensual stereotypes ($r_s > r_2$), and acquaintance (n).

overlap, there is a slight positive relationship between acquaintance and consensus. Interestingly, with high overlap and strong physical-appearance effects, consensus uniformly decreases with increasing acquaintance.

Figures 4.2 through 4.5 clearly show that the strength of the effect of acquaintance on consensus depends heavily on the overlap parameter (q). If there is high overlap, there is virtually no increase in consensus as acquaintance increases. Also, even if overlap is low, strong consensus about physical-appearance cues can lead to a relatively flat relationship between consensus and acquaintance. These results, though not supported by common sense, are supported by the longitudinal studies reviewed earlier in this chapter. Those studies reveal little or no relationship between consensus and acquaintance.

As acquaintance increases, the maximum limit of consensus, assuming no communication, is the degree to which meaning systems are shared. Whatever the number of acts, the limit for c is the correlation between act scale values. To return to Figures 4.2 through 4.5, all of the curves asymptote at .5, the value of r_2.

Both overlap and similar meaning systems drive consensus. So far, the consistency parameter has not been varied. The effect of consistency on consensus depends heavily on overlap. If overlap is perfect, then the level of consistency has little or no effect on consensus. However, if either there is not perfect overlap or the unique impression has a weight other than zero (more technically, $r_5 < r_2$), then as consistency increases, so does consensus. But if n is large and even if overlap is zero, consistency can be very small, yet consensus can be moderate.

This is illustrated in the top panel of Figure 4.6. It has been assumed that k, w, q, and a equal zero, and that $r_2 = .5$. Presumably, perceivers sample many target acts—probably hundreds. So in Figure 4.6, n varies from 1 to 500. Given the law of large numbers, low consistency can lead to moderate consensus. Recall that, given no overlap as acquaintance increases, consensus approaches r_2 (similar meaning systems) as long as there is some consistency. As consistency increases, consensus approaches r_2 more rapidly. So in Figure 4.6, for both $r_1 = .01$ and .10, c approaches .5 (the value of r_2), but it does so more rapidly when $r_1 = .10$. The model can then explain why studies of behavioral consistency at the act level show very low correlations (often nonsignificant ones), whereas consensus between perceivers appears to be moderate. Consistency can be extremely low, but because perceivers sample hundreds of acts, they can agree at a moderate level.

In the bottom panel of Figure 4.6, the effects of unique impression and physical appearance are included in the model. It is assumed

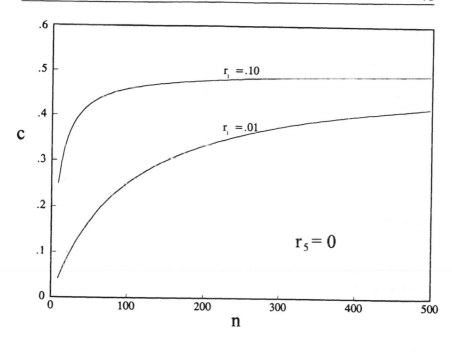

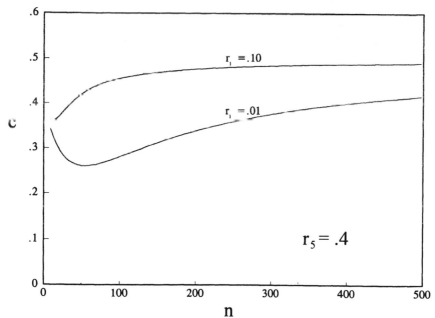

FIGURE 4.6. Consensus (c) as a function of consistency (r_1), consensual stereotypes (r_5), and acquaintance (n).

that $w = k = 5$ and that $r_3 = .8$, making $r_5 = .4$ and all other parameters as they are in the top panel. The presence of consensual physical-appearance information weakens the relationship between consensus and acquaintance when overlap is low, and makes it concave or bowl-like. Interestingly, the curves for two levels of consistency are nearly parallel when the effects of physical appearance are added to the model.

If acquaintance is high and there is no communication, then the other parameters have little influence on the level of consensus. The value of c approaches r_2, given that $r_1 > 0$. If $r_1 = 0$, then for large n, consensus approaches qr_2. Thus, given a high level of acquaintance, the level of consistency (as long as it is greater than zero) does not affect the level of consensus. Therefore, consensus is not determined very much by the level of consistency, especially for people who know each other well.

The "kernel of truth" parameter, or r_4, has relatively little effect on consensus. However, it has a dramatic effect on accuracy, which is discussed in Chapter 7.

When the communication parameter is positive, consensus is enhanced. As the communication parameter increases, the consensus correlation approaches unity. Large communication effects may obscure the effects of the other parameters. If, however, the communication parameter is negative (e.g., the perceivers dislike each other), then communication lowers consensus. It would seem that such "boomerang effects" (Abelson & Miller, 1967) are probably infrequent, because people are unlikely to communicate with those whom they dislike.

Summary

Under the condition of high overlap, there is little or no relationship between consensus and acquaintance. As overlap decreases, the relationship between consensus and acquaintance becomes more complex. If physical-appearance cues play an important role in perception and they are highly consensual, consensus initially declines in acquaintance and then later increases. If physical-appearance information is less important or its meaning is not consensual, then increasing acquaintance does lead to greater consensus.

Assuming no communication and some consistency, the upper limit of consensus is the parameter of similar meaning systems. If there is no consistency, then the upper limit is overlap times similar meaning systems. Consistency increases consensus only when both overlap and acquaintance are low. In general, overlap and similar meaning systems are more important parameters than are consistency and acquaintance.

General Discussion

The Low Level of Consensus

Commenting on essentially the same set of studies of consensus, Ross and Nisbett (1991) stated that the correlations "were not very high" (p. 99), whereas Kenrick and Funder (1988) asserted that "it is clear that the use of reliable rating scales leads to high agreement regarding a target's personality" (p. 25). Whether one considers the levels of consensus in Table 4.2 as high or low has become a controversial issue.

Two things can be said about the level of agreement. First, judges do agree with one another, especially when they have information about the target. Second, judges also disagree with one another; well over two-thirds of the variance represents disagreement. This section discusses why judges disagree and considers factors that may have led to an underestimation of the level of consensus.

Why Do Judges Disagree?

In WAM (Kenny, 1991), there are three different sources of disagreement in the rating of a target by two judges: nonoverlap, different meaning systems, and unique impression. "Nonoverlap" refers to the fact that the two judges see different target behaviors, and that is why they disagree. As can be seen by comparing the second and third rows of Table 4.2 (the one-on-one vs. the group studies), nonoverlap does substantially reduce the level of consensus. However, even when the judges see identical information, the level of consensus is not very impressive. Hence, the disagreement is probably attributable to other factors besides nonoverlap.

The second source of disagreement in WAM is different meaning systems. When judges see the same behavior, they may attach different meanings to it. Attribution theory emphasizes the fact that perceivers often give different meanings to the same behavior. Therefore, the biases that judges have may be rather idiosyncratic, in that different judges give very different meanings to the same behavior.

The third source of disagreement, which is not stimulus-based, is the use of unique impression or irrelevant and unshared information. For instance, a judge may be in a good mood, and so he or she may rate the target favorably. Although evidently judges form unique impressions of targets, it is difficult to disentangle the irrelevant-information explanation from the lack of shared meaning.

Is the Level of Consensus Underestimated?

Some might feel that the level of consensus has been seriously underestimated. Perhaps higher levels of consensus may appear in the literature because studies showing low levels of consensus are less likely to be published. Because all of the studies that could be located that met our strict methodological criteria were included in our review (Kenny et al., in press), some of the studies are unpublished. Although the level of consensus in our review is lower than that found in some studies using different designs and analysis strategies (Paulhus & Bruce, 1992), it is consistent with results of many other studies (e.g., John & Robins, 1993; Woodruffe, 1984).

It is important to realize that our estimates of consensus are conservative. Because most of the measures that were studied were single-item measures, they probably contained a great deal of error variance. In Chapter 5, it is estimated that about 45% of the variance in the ratings can be considered as error. Given such a value, the true levels of the proportion of target variance should be much larger when less error-laden measures are used.

In addition, even though about a .2 level of consensus was found in many studies, that does not imply that only 20% of the variance in peer ratings is reliable. In some rating studies, the same judges evaluate all the targets. With this design, the judge variance can be removed from the denominator. About 20% of the variance is judge variance (see Chapter 5), and so for this type of design, there would be about a 25% increase in consensus. Moreover, the percentage-of-target-variance measure of consensus states the reliability of a single judge. Most rating studies use more than one rater. With the present measure of consensus, the Spearman–Brown prophecy formula (Nunnally, 1967) can be used to forecast the agreement between two groups of raters. For instance, if the proportion of target variance is .2, then the proportion of target variance of the mean averaged over four raters should be .5. So the proportion of target variance of a group of judges may be substantial.

Finally, all of the studies included in our survey used college students. It seems reasonable to believe that research using a less homogeneous, more representative sample would find larger levels of consensus. Support for this contention is provided by Borkenau and Liebler (1992), who found enhanced levels of consensus at zero acquaintance when a community sample was used.

Greater Consensus for Extroversion

The review has shown that Extroversion operates very differently from the other Big Five factors. Generally, Extroversion shows the highest level of consensus. Other studies have also pointed to greater consensus in the rating of Extroversion as opposed to other traits (Funder & Dobroth, 1987; Park & Judd, 1989). The review indicates that Extroversion information is picked up very quickly, in that consensus is relatively high at zero acquaintance. Alternatively, it could be argued that there exist strong cultural stereotypes that do have a "kernel of truth."

These early impressions of Extroversion are remarkably stable over time. Table 4.5 presents the over-time correlation from zero acquaintance to a postinteraction rating from four studies. The table clearly shows that there is high stability in the Extroversion judgments made at zero acquaintance. Not only are Extroversion judgments made at zero acquaintance stable, they are also valid. A recent study (Levesque & Kenny, 1993) indicates that consensual judgments made at zero acquaintance predict subsequent behaviors of the target (see Chapter 7).

Interestingly, consensus on Extroversion drops in one on one studies (see Table 4.2, and see Kenny et al., 1992, Study 2). Extroversion is revealed more clearly in group interactions than it is in dyadic interactions. A likely part of the reason for this is the norm for equal participation in two-person interactions. Extroversion may be more relevant for group than for dyadic interaction.

What parameter within WAM leads to the higher levels of consensus for Extroversion? There are two potential candidates. First, the parameter of similar meaning systems may be greater for Extroversion than it is for other Big Five factors. Evidence that Extroversion is more observable than other factors (Funder & Dobroth, 1987; Park & Judd, 1989) is consistent with this point of view. Second, target

TABLE 4.5. Stability of the Target Effect of Extroversion beyond Zero Acquaintance

Study	Stability
Kenny et al. (1992), Study 2	.89
Kenny et al. (1992), Study 3	.72
Albright et al. (1988), Study 1	.86[a]
Malloy (1987a)	.69[a]

Note. Adapted from Kenny et al. (in press). Copyright 1994 by the American Psychological Association. Adapted by permission.
[a]Averaged across two times.

behavior may be more consistent for Extroversion than it is for the other factors. Surprisingly, Park et al. (1994) found no evidence that Extroversion had greater similar meaning systems or consistency than the other factors. However, Park et al. used written, not visual, stimuli.

Consensus and Acquaintance

The cross-sectional studies included in our review (Kenny et al., in press) point to increased consensus with increased interaction for all factors except Extroversion. However, the longitudinal studies show little or no evidence of such a trend. The longitudinal results probably present a more realistic picture of the relationship between consensus and acquaintance. There are three reasons why the longitudinal results may be more credible.

First, it is well known that trends from cross-sectional studies can be very misleading. In a cross-sectional study, different groups of people are being compared on different variables with different formats in different settings. Longitudinal comparisons are typically (though not always) more valid than cross-sectional comparisons.

In addition, in the cross-sectional studies reviewed, communication effects posited by WAM were probably stronger in the long-term acquaintance studies than in the short-term acquaintance studies, because in many of the latter there was no opportunity for communication. The strongest piece of evidence supporting a relationship between acquaintance and consensus is the comparison between short-term interactions and long-term interactions. Except for Extroversion, there is impressive evidence of greater consensus among those who were acquainted longer. But the long-term acquaintance results are probably biased by communication. Recall that all of the long-term acquaintance studies were residential; judges probably discussed with one another the personalities of mutual acquaintances, and that communication may well have led to greater consensus. We (Kenny & Kashy, in press) have found greater consensus between friends than acquaintances, a result that indicates a communication effect. However, the size of that effect is small. Although we need more controlled studies to measure the effect of communication on consensus, these recent results seem to indicate that communication may explain some of the increase in consensus from short-term to long-term acquaintance.

Lastly, the heightened consensus in the long-term studies probably reflects qualitative differences in information available to the subjects. Again, the long-term acquaintance studies were all residential studies, whereas the short-term acquaintance studies were laboratory or classroom studies. Clearly, a person can obtain much more information in a residential setting than in either of the other two settings. Thus, the laboratory and classroom settings may have constrained the targets' behavior, and that may be why there appears to be more consensus in the long-term versus the short-term acquaintance studies.

So what is the relationship between acquaintance and consensus? For Extroversion, there is no evidence that increasing acquaintance leads to greater consensus. For the other factors, there is some evidence supporting the view that getting to know the target better does lead to greater consensus, though this evidence is not conclusive. As is predicted by WAM, even for these factors, there is not a strong relationship between consensus and acquaintance.

Future Research

Although a great many studies have been reviewed, there are nonetheless substantial gaps in the literature. Two different types of studies are essential. First, more residential studies are needed. The review in this chapter included just five such studies, and only one was longitudinal. These studies should focus on non-Extroversion traits, and they should try to get measurements as early as possible in the acquaintance process. It may well be that after 1 week of interaction, the level of consensus will have peaked. Longitudinal studies of people living together deserve a high priority.

Second, only 1 of the 32 studies was a longitudinal study across days of one-on-one interactions. A laboratory study that repeatedly brought people to interact in dyads would provide important information. Because the interactions would be dyadic, communication effects and overlap effects would probably be eliminated. Traits studied should not be those for which there are strong consensual stereotypes. If there are stereotypes, then the likely shape of the relationship between consensus and acquaintance is concave, first decreasing and then increasing.

Conclusion

We (Kenny et al., in press) have found the highest level of consensus for the following two conditions: when the factor is Extroversion, and when perceiver and target are highly acquainted. Research efforts need to concentrate on why perceivers agree so little with one another. Much of person perception is unique—a topic that is also discussed in

Chapters 5 and 10. A blending of laboratory studies in which the stimuli are under experimental control and non-laboratory studies is needed.

Surprisingly, especially for Extroversion and Conscientiousness, there are nontrivial levels of agreement at zero acquaintance; this result is consistent with work by Ambady and Rosenthal (1992) and Berry (1990). Evidently the stereotypes about these factors are potent and consensual.

The most surprising result is the weak increase in consensus as a function of acquaintance. The expectation of greater acquaintance leading to greater consensus received limited support in our review. This result is no longer surprising, given a theoretical model predicting that consensus does not always increase with increased acquaintance. It is shown in Chapter 7 that although acquaintance may not lead to increased consensus, it should lead to increased target accuracy.

This chapter has focused mainly on the relationship between consensus and acquaintance. In the process other factors have been discussed, but the central focus has always been acquaintance and consensus. Many other questions about consensus could have been discussed. For example, John and Robins (1993) have examined whether there is more or less consensus for socially desirable traits. The Kenny and Kashy (in press) study has looked at whether close friends share the same view of a target to a greater extent than acquaintances. Flink and Park (1991) have discussed whether increasing the specificity of the rating and the outcome dependency increases consensus. Unfortunately, space and time are limited, and a full consideration of these consensus questions is just not possible.

Consensus is not only intrinsically important, but it is a prerequisite for many of the other questions in interpersonal perception. For instance, self–other agreement, to be discussed in Chapter 9, presumes consensus. Consensus is also presumed in the study of target accuracy (Chapter 7), meta-accuracy (Chapter 8), and reciprocity at the individual level of analysis (Chapter 6). Thus, the results from this chapter lay the groundwork for the analysis in subsequent chapters.

Notes

1. In one study (Kenny & DePaulo, 1990), the dyads were asymmetric: A group of three interviewers questioned three applicants one at a time. Because of the asymmetry in the dyads, it did not seem sensible to consider the research as a single study, and so it was separated into two different studies. There was also some overlap in one other study: The people in the three-wave Malloy (1987a) longitudinal study represented 24% of the people from Study 3 of Albright, Kenny, and Malloy (1988).

2. As in Kenny (1991), it is assumed here that the correlation of perceiver 1's scale value for A_1 with perceiver 2's scale value for A_2 is equal to $r_1 r_2$. Also to simplify, the correlation of s_{1P} with s_{22} is equal to $r_3 r_4$. These assumptions are relaxed in Appendix C.

3. For the case in which $r_5 = r_2$ (Figure 4.3), it is assumed that $w = 2$, $k = 1$, and $r_3 = .625$, and so $r_5 = .5$. For the case in which $r_5 < r_2$ (Figure 4.4), it is assumed that $w = .5$, $k = 2.179$, and $r_3 = .6$, and so $r_5 = .03$. Finally, for the case in which $r_5 > r_2$ (Figure 4.5), it is assumed that $w = 2.179$, $k = .5$, and $r_3 = .75$, and so $r_5 = .7125$. In all cases, the combined weight of the physical-appearance information and the unique-impression information (i.e., $w^2 + k^2$) is 5.

Chapter 5

UNIQUENESS

As reviewed in the past two chapters, within the Social Relations Model (SRM) there are two sources of individual differences in the perceptions of others: perceiver and target effects. However, there are clearly relational aspects in social perception. For instance, people view their lovers and their enemies in a way that no one else does. Uniqueness seems to be a major component in the perception of people. This chapter considers the uniqueness, or, as it is referred to within SRM, the relationship effect in other-perception.

The chapter begins by showing that uniqueness is an important component in other-perception. Considered next is the relationship between uniqueness in other-perception and affect. A discussion then follows of the sources or explanations of uniqueness in interpersonal perception: different information, different meaning, unique impression, and mathematical specification. Finally, the relationship between uniqueness and acquaintance is considered.

The "relationship effect" in SRM refers to the extent to which a perceiver's view of a target cannot be explained by perceiver and target effects. It represents what remains after the individual-level effects have been removed. The relationship effect consists of the "leftovers." In the rating process, as in any measurement process, there are random, theoretically meaningless sources of variance that are referred to as "measurement errors." Because the relationship component is what remains after perceiver and target effects have been removed, measurement error is contained in the relationship component. If there were only a single measure of a perception, then the relationship variance and hence uniqueness would be overstated, because error would be confounded with relationship effects (Ingraham & Wright, 1986).

To separate relationship from error, it is necessary to have multiple measures of the trait being assessed. As an example, consider the measurement of Extroversion. Two possible measures of Extroversion might be how sociable and how outgoing the perceivers see the targets as being. With multiple measures, it is possible to correlate what is "left over" in both measures, and this correlation represents real relationship variance. (It would be an "intrapersonal relationship" correlation as described in Chapter 2.) So in this chapter, to separate relationship from error, all measures of relationship variance employ multiple measures of the variable of interest. The requirement of multiple replications greatly reduces the number of studies that can be used, but it should substantially enhance the validity of the conclusions that are drawn.

These multiple measures of the variable, or "replications," can be obtained either by employing different measures of the theoretical construct or by using the same measure at multiple time points. Each of these procedures has its own advantages and disadvantages. It seems likely that the use of different measures somewhat overstates the amount of relationship variance, in that the errors of measurement may be correlated across measures. Using over-time measures probably understates the amount of relationship variance, because change is treated as error. The ideal procedure is to use different measures over a very short time (i.e., a short enough time that change is unlikely to have occurred). However, this strategy is not generally practical.

Uniqueness versus Assimilation and Consensus

Table 5.1 presents the results from the variance partitioning in 10 studies. These studies contain a range of acquaintance levels and types of variables. Presented for each study are the perceiver variances, or assimilation; the target variances, or consensus; and the relationship variances, or uniqueness. Not included in the table is the error variance, which equals 1 minus the sum of the three.

Across the 10 studies, the amount of relationship variance averages to .197. There is more relationship variance than there is target variance, both on average and for 8 of the 10 studies. So the expectation is for greater relationship variance than target variance, and for nearly as much relationship variance as perceiver variance.

Even more impressive than the average level of relationship variance is how stable it is. Note that uniqueness ranges from a low of .13 (a zero-acquaintance study) to a high of .29; target variances are much more variable. The last row of Table 5.1 presents the standard deviation, which indexes variability; it clearly documents that uniqueness does not vary all that much from study to study. Relationship variance is always present at a respectable level.

The medians in Table 5.1 can be used to develop a general

TABLE 5.1. Variance Partitioning of Other-Perception

Study	Relative variance		
	Assimilation	Consensus	Uniqueness
Albright, Kenny, & Malloy (1988), Study 3	.13	.08	.13
Chapdelaine, Kenny, & LaFontana (in press)	.16	.11	.18
Kenny, Horner, Kashy, & Chu (1992), Study 2, wave 1	.25	.04	.22
Kenny et al. (1992), Study 3, wave 1	.25	.15	.18
DePaulo, Kenny, Hoover, Webb, & Oliver (1987)	.37	.07	.18
Kenny & DePaulo (1990), applicant	.19	.35	.15
Hallmark & Kenny (1989)	.20	.23	.29
Levesque (1990)	.18	.18	.20
Malloy & Janowski (1992)	.06	.45	.24
Shechtman & Kenny (in press)	.25	.11	.20
Mean	.20	.18	.20
Median	.19	.13	.19
Standard deviation	.08	.13	.04

formulation of the sources of variance in other-perception. It suggests a "20–20 and 15–45" rule: The expectation is about 20% for perceiver variance, about 20% for relationship variance, about 15% for target variance, and about 45% for error variance. Of course, this is just a general rule, and specific cases may be very different. For instance, in Chapter 4 it has been found that Extroversion usually accounts for more than 20% of the variance. This 20–20 and 15–45 rule is again discussed in the final chapter of the book. In summary, uniqueness is as important as assimilation, and more important than consensus.

Affect versus Other-Perception

It would seem that affect, more so than other-perception, is primarily a relational phenomenon. The notion of "love at first sight," and the idea that liking is not so much a property of the target but rather reflects something *between* people, suggest that liking or affect is primarily relational. This section focuses on two questions. First, is there relatively more relationship variance in affect than there is in other-perception? Second, what is the correlation between affect and other-perception at the relationship level? The first question establishes the fact that affect is primarily relational, and the second concerns the relative independence of affect and other-perception.

Common sense is not very helpful in establishing whether affect or liking is primarily relational. On the one hand, there is a sense that liking is very idiosyncratic; on the other, people *believe* that if they like someone, then everyone should like that person (Chapdelaine, Kenny, & LaFontana, in press). How often are young people surprised that significant others (parents and best friends) do not like their boyfriends or girlfriends?

In terms of human evolution, it would seem to be adaptive that affect is relational. If everyone wanted to be friends with the same person, and if everyone wanted to have the same opposite-sex person for a spouse, conflict would be the rule of human relationships. If affect were relational (and, as is seen in the next chapter, also reciprocal), pair bonding would be facilitated, and conflict about mate and friendship choice would be reduced. Although it is largely a matter of speculation, there may be biological forces that incline humans to form idiosyncratic attractions.

Table 5.2 presents the proportion of variance attributable to relationship in studies of traits and affect. The requirement of at least two measures of the trait and two of affect greatly limits the number of studies. Despite these limitations, Table 5.2 clearly shows that relationship variance is much greater for affect than for other-perception. As seen in the table, there is nearly twice as much relationship variance in affect as there is in trait ratings.

Elsewhere (Kenny, 1994), looking only at affect, I also arrived at the conclusion that about 40% of affect is relational. Table 5.3 presents that summary. The table shows that about 20% of the

TABLE 5.2. Trait and Affect Relationship Variance and Correlation

Study	Relative variance		Correlation
	Trait	Affect	
Kashy (1988)	.21	.48	.48
Malloy & Janowski (1992)	.24	.32	.52
Chapdelaine et al. (in press)	.18	.38	.76
Montgomery (1984)	.22	.38	.84
Mean	.21	.39	.65

TABLE 5.3. Variance Partitioning for Liking

Study	Perceiver	Target	Relationship
First encounters: One-on-one			
Burleson (1983)	.20	.28	.32
Kenny & Bernstein (1982)	.00	.05	.55
First encounters: Groups			
Dabbs & Ruback (1987)	.30	.13	.37
Kashy (1988)	.32	.06	.44
Park & Flink (1989)	.36	.11	.38
Long-term acquaintance			
Burleson (1983)	.17	.18	.30
Curry & Emerson (1970)	.15	.12	.41
Malloy & Albright (1990)	.10	.00	.50
Newcomb (1961)	—[a]	.41	.50
Wright, Ingraham, & Blackmer (1985)	.05	.16	.30
Median	.17	.13	.38

Note. Adapted from Kenny (1994). Copyright 1994 by Lawrence Erlbaum Associates, Inc. Adapted by permission.
[a]Because ranks were used, perceiver variance cannot be computed.

variance of liking is at the level of the perceiver, about 10% at the level of the target, and about 40% at the level of the relationship.

Table 5.2 also presents the correlation between trait and affect at the relationship level. These correlations are consistently positive and average to about .65. The relationship is a disattenuated correlation, and so it is a forecast of what the correlation would be if there were no error in the liking measure. If the view is taken that affect causes other-perception, then about 40% of the variance in trait ratings at the relationship level is attributable to affect. A person's unique view of a target overlaps considerably with, but is different from, the feeling that the person has toward the target.

Park and Flink (1989) showed that the correlation between affect and trait judgments depends on the trait being judged. In their study, the correlation for Extroversion (their Factor 1) was .52, and for the other traits the correlation was .78. Affect correlated more highly with less observable traits.

Does the association between affect and trait judgments increase as the perceiver and target become more acquainted? The studies in Table 5.3 are ordered by how long the people knew each other. Interestingly, the results clearly show that affect and trait judgments become increasingly more positively correlated. Park and Flink (1989) also reported over-time correlations between trait judgments and liking; they too found an increasing correlation over time. In one longitudinal study, Albright-Malloy (1988) reported that affect and trait judgments became increasingly differentiated over time. However, Albright-Malloy did not have multiple measures of affect, and so her results are somewhat problematic.

In conclusion, affect contains nearly twice as much uniqueness as trait ratings. In sum, the evidence supports the view that affect is closely linked to trait judgments at the level of the relationship, and that the association increases with acquaintance. Later in the chapter, I discuss the causal direction of the liking–cognition relationship.

Interpretation of the Relationship Effect

Although it hardly requires proof that there is uniqueness in social perception data, it is not clear what the meaning of the relationship effect is. This section considers four different explanations of the relationship effect in other-perception. Three of these explanations draw on the Weighted-Average Model (WAM) presented in Chapter 4. In WAM, there are three reasons why two perceivers may disagree about the standing of a target on a trait: different information, different meaning systems, and different unique impressions. The fourth explanation of the relationship effect is mathematical: The mathematical model presumed by SRM is faulty.

The Relationship Effect as Different Information

Two perceivers may judge a target differently because the two perceivers have been exposed to different information about the target. Murderers are seen as upright people by their own parents, but the parents of their victims see them as totally reprehensible. A murderer's parents saw the murderer as a helpless child, whereas the victim's parents know only of the brutal act that brought about their child's death. Thus, these two sets of parents see the murderer differently because they draw on different sources of information when they evaluate him or her.

Therefore, it is reasonable to expect that when people use different information, there should be more relationship variance and less target variance. Evidence reported in Chapter 4 does indeed show that there is more target variance when people use different information, but is there less relationship variance?

Table 5.4 presents the absolute relationship variances from one of our studies (Study 2 by Kenny, Horner, Kashy, & Chu, 1992). That study compared group judgment to one-on-one judgments. However, it should be noted that the group judgments were made at zero acquaintance, and so perceivers in the one-on-one context had more information. As seen in Table 5.4, relationship variances are larger after one-on-one interaction than at zero acquaintance. These results support the view that one source of relationship variance is different information.

Not surprisingly, having different stimulus information results in greater uniqueness in perceptions. But this is, in some sense, a false uniqueness, in that the target's behavior is really different; this is why the two perceivers have very different impressions. The next two explanations are much more interesting, because in these explanations the perceiver is exposed to the same set of target behaviors.

The Relationship Effect as Different Meaning Systems

Even when two perceivers observe exactly the same set of behaviors, they may interpret those behaviors quite differently. A person looks across the room and notices that a second person is staring back at him or her. In this situation, one person may think that the second person has friendly intentions, whereas another may think that the second person has evil intentions. Very often the same cue is given a different meaning by different people. A man's gentle squeeze of a woman's hand may be seen as a sign of affection and caring by him and as a form of sexual harassment by her.

There are three very different ways to understand how acts can be given different meanings: attribution, stories, and culture. All three of these explanations are interrelated, yet it is useful to separate them.

TABLE 5.4. Relationship Variances for Group and Dyadic Judgments from Kenny et al. (1992), Study 2

Factor	Group	Dyadic
Extroversion	.26	.47
Agreeableness	.23	.12
Conscientiousness	.10	.14
Emotional Stability	.07	.24
Culture	.00	.14
Mean	.13	.22

Attribution

Social psychologists have long known that people interpret the same information differently, and over the last 20 or so years, they have extensively studied the attribution process. The attribution question concerns, in part, when is it that behavior is seen as emanating from the person or from the situation. If different attributions are made, the same behavior is explained in different ways. A slap in the face can be viewed as a direct personal affront or as an unfortunate accident.

Social psychologists have enumerated many factors that change people's attributions. Because standard books on person perception (Jones, 1990; Schneider, Hastorf, & Ellsworth, 1979; Zebrowitz, 1990) extensively detail these biases, only a few are discussed in this text. First, if a person is similar to a target, the target is seen as less responsible for his or her bad behaviors and more responsible for his or her good behaviors. This attributional bias, called "defensive attribution" (Burger, 1981), implies that people tend to make more positive trait judgments about those who are similar to them.

A second factor is "personalism" (Jones, 1990). If an action affects the perceiver, he or she is more likely to infer that the behavior is caused by the target. So if Heidi sees Zelda step on someone else's toe, Heidi may think it is an accident and not Zelda's fault. But if Zelda steps on Heidi's toe, then Heidi is likely to think that Zelda is clumsy and awkward.

Social psychologists have studied a myriad of factors that lead people to make different attributions. If the reason for uniqueness in other-perception is attribution, then it must be that attributions are fundamentally idiosyncratic. That is, although it is possible to catalog a myriad of factors that lead to attributions, people may make different attributions spontaneously and without any clear reason. So if two people observe the same behavior, they may interpret the behavior very differently because they made different attributions. Contrary to current thinking in social psychology, the attributional process may not be a set of systematic biases, but rather a set of idiosyncratic biases.

Stories or Narratives

Person perception can be conceptualized as more than just a simple translation of behavioral information into trait judgments. Solomon Asch, generally recognized as the founder of the scientific study of person perception, viewed person perception as a Gestalt or holistic process. According to Asch (1946), the perceiver does not combine behavioral information by using some mathematical function (e.g., as is assumed by WAM); rather, the perceiver integrates the information in an active and complex manner. The perceiver tries to create a story or a narrative to explain behavioral information. If person perception is viewed from this Gestalt perspective, it is not surprising that different perceivers give different meanings to the same information, because each perceiver concocts a different story.

The task that a person faces in interpersonal perception can be viewed as similar to the task faced by a detective in solving a murder. The detective assembles the facts and develops a coherent story that connects those facts. As readers of murder mysteries know, the same facts often lend themselves to multiple versions. Pennington and Hastie (1991) have described the process by which juries come to a verdict as one of "collective story construction." Person perceivers may engage in such a process. Recently, several researchers in person perception have begun to explore the story or narrative approach. Park, DeKay, and Kraus (1994) have used the term "person model"; Read and Miller (1993) have referred to "mental models"; and Fiske (1993) has discussed "narratives."

This view of person perception requires a radical alteration of the model of perception proposed in Chapter 4, WAM. The story model implicitly assumes that people select a rather small set of behaviors to construct a theory about what the person is like. The remaining behaviors are assimilated into this image. From the point of view of WAM, in forming an impression, a perceiver places much more weight on some behaviors than on others. Because different perceivers pick different behaviors, the impressions of different perceivers are highly idiosyncratic. WAM could be modified to allow for differential weighting of behavioral information, but still the story or narrative model is a qualitatively different model from WAM, with its piecemeal integration of information.

Culture

There is yet another way in which two perceivers may arrive at different meanings: They may be members of different cultures. Culture by definition provides people with meaning systems, in that it provides a way of linking behaviors to particular trait judgments. The linkage structure between behaviors and traits may be quite different for members of different cultures. As reviewed in Chapter 4, anthropologists have recently begun to conceptualize consensus as an index of culture.

Culture also can be defined more narrowly than it usually is. For instance, Tannen (1990) suggests that men and women are members of different cultures. For instance, she argues that in conversation, women are interested in intimacy and men in power. SRM can be used to document and quantify the extent to which different groups of people have different meaning systems. Procedures for doing so are to be discussed in the "Mathematical Specification" section of this chapter.

The Relationship Effect as Idiosyncratic Perception

In a third explanation, the uniqueness in the perception is entirely in the mind of the perceiver. In the model described in Chapter 4, the "unique impression" represents aspects of perception that are perceiver-based and are not based on the behavior of the target. For instance, a woman may think that a man is intelligent not because of anything he has done, but because she is in love with him.

As shown in Table 5.2, there is a strong correlation between affect and other-perception at the relationship level. A person's unique views of others are colored by how much the person likes others.[1]

An alternate view is that affect is determined by how the target is viewed. That is, the correlation between affect and trait judgment reflects the influence of cognition on affect: If people know positive things about a target, they evaluate that target more favorably. The dominant theory of social attitudes, Fishbein and Ajzen's (1975) theory of reasoned action, takes the point of view that beliefs lead to evaluations and not vice versa. Alternatively, Zajonc (1980) has argued that affect is primary. Certainly causation can go both ways (from affect to cognition and vice versa), but currently there does not exist a definitive study documenting the relative preponderance of causation in interpersonal perception.

Some traits are more affectively laden than others; for example, judgments of Extroversion are less tied to affect than are judgments of Conscientiousness, Culture, Emotional Stability, and that portion of Agreeableness not tied to sociability. It seems likely that Agreeableness would be the factor most closely tied to affect.

Other factors besides affect color the unique impression. In particular, the impression of a target may also be caused by mood. When people are in a good mood, they may evaluate targets more favorably than they do when they are in a bad mood. Actually, the interrelation between mood and person perception is quite complex (Forgas, 1992). Further research on the relationship between mood and person perception is warranted.

Mathematical Specification

Pseudo-relationship effects can emerge if the combination of perceiver and target effects does not operate in a simple additive fashion, as is assumed by SRM. There are four particular types of nonadditivity that are worrisome: the multiplicative functional form; the single-cue, differential-weight model; the multiple-cue, equal-weight model; and the multiple-cue, differential-weight model. Unfortunately, most of the material in this section is speculative. That is, there have not been systematic attempts to verify empirically these alternate mathematical speculations.

Multiplicative Functional Form

In the first possible mathematical specification, perceiver and target effects do not add together, as they are assumed to do in SRM; rather, they multiply together. So the functional form is multiplicative and not additive. Consider, for instance, a measure of social acuity. The measure is how accurately perceiver A judges target B. It is probably more reasonable in this context to argue that perceiver and target effects do not add, but rather multiply. For instance, if either the perceiver has no ability or the target does not provide sufficient information, the perceiver must necessarily be inaccurate. Accuracy is the mathematical product of perceiver ability and target expressivity. The simple solution to the problem of multiplicative functional form is to employ a logarithmic transformation. If the model is multiplicative, then a logarithmic transformation turns the model into an additive model.[2]

The next three mathematical models presume that interpersonal perception is not guided by the same process for all people. If a process is "nomological," all people operate by the same set of laws; if a process is "ipsative," different rules describe the behavior of different people. The three models to be discussed below view interpersonal perception from an ipsative perspective. People may use the same cues to make judgments about targets, but they may combine those cues in different ways. In a sense, the models to be discussed represent a mathematical specification of what is meant by "different meaning systems," particularly in connection with culture. In essence, these methods provide a way of discovering different "cultures" of perceivers.

Single-Cue, Differential-Weight Model

The simplest ipsative model is one in which people use the same information in making judgments, but some people weight that information more heavily than do others. Some perceivers may be quite sensitive to the stimulus information, whereas other perceivers may not be. The expected pattern of results implied by this type of model

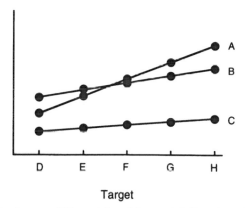

Target

FIGURE 5.1. Single-cue, differential-weight model. Perceiver A is the most sensitive, and C is the least sensitive.

is illustrated in Figure 5.1. There are five targets and three perceivers in the figure. Perceiver *Alex,* or A, is quite sensitive; *Bob,* or B, is less so; and *Carol,* or C, has virtually no sensitivity. The personality psychologist Douglas Jackson (1972) has postulated just such a model, which he has called a model of "inferential accuracy."

Standard SRM assumes that all judges are equally sensitive. SRM requires that the three lines in Figure 5.1 be parallel. When the lines are not parallel as in Figure 5.1, there is, in essence, more target variance for perceiver A than for perceiver C.

As reviewed in Chapter 3, numerous theorists have posited that some people use certain traits more than others. The personality psychologist George Kelly (1955) referred to "personal constructs"; the social psychologists Higgins and Bargh (1987) have used the term "chronicity"; and the social psychologist Markus (1977) has proposed the construct of being "schematic" versus "aschematic" on a trait. All these notions imply differential sensitivity.

There are other ways of explaining the differences in slope that have nothing to do with "sensitivity." First, it may be that the more "sensitive" perceivers are engaging in more, not less, stereotyping (i.e., using physical-appearance information) than those who are less "sensitive." Second, it may be that the more "sensitive" perceivers adopt a response set that involves using the entire range of possible response alternatives, whereas the less "sensitive" use a narrower range. Thus, researchers should not necessarily equate steeper slopes, as in Figure 5.1, with greater social sensitivity.

Multiple-Cue, Equal-Weight Model

A second ipsative model of person perception is the following: There are two cues, and some perceivers exclusively use one cue, whereas others use the second cue.[3] So perceivers can be grouped into discrete types. For instance, in judgments of physical attractiveness, some may exclusively examine the face, whereas others may examine the rest of the body. If different cues are used, then perceivers have different definitions for the trait. They are, in a sense, members of different cultures.

If there is such a process, then it may be possible to uncover it by the following procedure. The researcher measures how similar the judgments are between every pair of perceivers. So there should be a measure of the consensus in the judgments of a common set of targets between each pair of perceivers. If there are two cultures, it follows that two groups or clusters of perceivers should emerge. If two perceivers are members of the same culture, there should be a fair amount of agreement or consensus in their ratings. But if two members are in different cultures, there should be much less agreement. There exist several statistical methods (e.g., cluster analysis or Q factor analysis) that can be used to discover the two rating groups.

Once the researcher has classified perceivers into cultures, the researcher should examine the targets to learn what were the different cues that the two groups used. So, to return to the physical-attractiveness example, one group of perceivers prefers targets with attractive faces and the other group prefers targets with attractive bodies. Basically, the researcher takes a cue variable (e.g., facial attractiveness) and sees whether it differentially predicts the target effects of the two subgroups. If an SRM analysis is carried out separately on each of the two groups of perceivers, there should be much more target variance and less relationship variance (i.e., more consensus and less uniqueness) than if both groups of perceivers are combined in one analysis.

Multiple-Cue, Differential-Weight Model

The preceding model presupposes that the perceivers are using different cues to judge behavior. An alternate view is that people use the same set of cues, but in somewhat different amounts. To use a metaphor, people may be using the same recipe in interpersonal perception, but they combine the ingredients in somewhat different proportions. Consider a case in which perceivers are asked to rate targets on aggressiveness. It seems likely that rated aggression depends on two important behavioral cues: verbal and physical aggression. Perceivers may differ in how much these two factors are weighted. Some perceivers may place greater weight on verbal aggression, whereas others may place more importance on physical aggression.

Consider the graph in Figure 5.2. The horizontal axis represents how important a perceiver thinks physical aggression is. The vertical axis represents how important a perceiver thinks verbal aggression is. In the graph there are three different perceivers. John thinks that both physical and verbal aggressions are important; Michael thinks that physical aggression is more important than verbal aggression; and Philip thinks that verbal aggression is more important than physical aggression. When it is said that a perceiver "thinks" that one form of aggression is more important than another, this does not mean necessarily that the perceiver *consciously* knows that he thinks one is more important than the other, but that the pattern in his ratings implies that he *implicitly* thinks this way.

To discover whether people differentially weight stimulus information, the similarity between every pair of perceivers is first computed. (A standard measure of profile similarity is the sum, across targets, of squared differences between a pair of perceivers. Before the difference is computed, the mean rating of each perceiver is usually subtracted.) Perceivers who use nearly identical weighting schemes should have very similar judgment profiles, and those who use different weighting schemes should have very different profiles. Individual-difference multidimensional scaling (INDSCAL; Jones, 1983) can be used to estimate these differences in importance. As with the model in the preceding section, it is necessary to examine the targets to understand the cues or features that are being differentially weighted. Park and Flink (1989) used a more conventional analysis strategy to

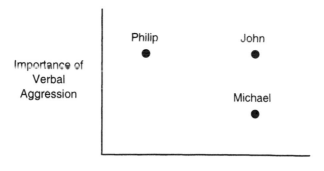

FIGURE 5.2. Differential importance of two cues in the rating process.

examine the differential weighting of two factors to determine affective judgments.

Actually, the two previous models are special cases of the two-cue, differential-weight model. If the one-cue, differential-weight model were correct, then the INDSCAL analysis would yield a single dimension on which individuals vary. If the two-cue, equal-weight model were true, then the INDSCAL analysis would yield two dimensions, but some people would use one and other people would use the second. So in Figure 5.2, there would be points for Philip and Michael and not for John.

Summary of Explanations

Four very different explanations have been put forth about the meaning of the relationship effect in other-perception. First, there is the somewhat trivial point that uniqueness may result when two perceivers are exposed to different target behaviors. Second, and most likely, perceivers may disagree because they attach different meanings to the target's behaviors. These different meaning systems may be related to differences in attributions, story construction, or culture. Third, the perceivers may disagree because they use nonbehavioral information (e.g., mood or liking) to evaluate the target. Fourth, different mathematical specifications are possible. It may be that perceivers are using different cues in evaluating targets, or that they are using the same cues but weighting them in different ways.

Acquaintance

In this section, the relative level of uniqueness as a function of acquaintance is considered, as well as the stability of the relationship effect or the over-time correlation.

Level of Uniqueness as a Function of Acquaintance

It is not obvious what the association between acquaintance and uniqueness should be. One could argue that it takes time to create relationships, and thus that with greater acquaintance there should be more relationship variance and so greater uniqueness. Alternatively, it could be argued that initial impressions are inadequate representations of the person, and that over time different people's impressions of a target converge. That is, as people get to know a target, they begin to know the target's true personality. These two different approaches conceptualize acquaintance in very different ways. The first approach looks at acquaintance as providing an opportunity for a deeper, closer relationship; thus acquaintance serves as a rough indicator for the quality of the relationship. The second approach treats acquaintance quantitatively: Getting to know a target resembles data analysis, and a perceiver is merely "gathering more data" as he or she gets to know the target.

So the qualitative model predicts increasing relationship variance as a function of acquaintance, whereas the quantitative model predicts decreasing relationship variance as a function of acquaintance. The two theories can be integrated as follows: The quantitative model is accurate during the early stages of acquaintance, and so with increasing acquaintance there should be decreasing relationship variance. But as a perceiver and a target come to know each other well, there is a qualitative shift, and interpersonal perception becomes more idiosyncratic. Thus, the relationship between acquaintance and uniqueness is curvilinear.

Surprisingly, there is not much evidence that the relationship variance changes to any great extent as a function of acquaintance. In fact, the two major studies of differences in relationship variance as a function of acquaintance found no confirming evidence. Park and Judd (1989) investigated college students who were initially strangers and who interviewed each other on four consecutive days; there was no evidence in this study of increasing uniqueness over time. We (Kenny & Kashy, in press) estimated relationship variance for friends and acquaintances. Contrary to our expectations, there was no difference in relationship variance in the two groups.

Although the evidence is skimpy, the following theoretical explanation is offered. Perhaps the effects of the qualitative model (which predicts increasing relationship variance as a function of acquaintance) and the quantitative model (which predicts decreasing relationship variance) operate simultaneously and not at different times, and so the net effect is to cancel each other out. This is one area where more research is clearly needed.

Stability of the Relationship Effect over Time

An important question is the stability of the relationship effect over time. Is Zelda's unique view of Heidi changeable or permanent? First considered is the transition from zero acquaintance to initial acquaint-

TABLE 5.5. Stability of Relationship Effect from Zero Acquaintance

Factor	Kenny et al. (1992), Study 2	Kenny et al. (1992), Study 3	Malloy (1987a)
Extroversion	.23	.19	.22
Agreeableness	.54	.38	.16
Conscientiousness	−.01	##	##
Emotional Stability	.12	.56	##
Culture	##	##	##

Note. ## = insufficient variance to compute correlation.

ance. Table 5.5 presents the stability correlations of the relationship effect across three different studies. The correlation is computed only if the relationship effect explains at least 10% of the variance at both times. Across the three studies, it is seen that there is relatively little stability in the relationship effect. The average correlation is only .27.

Once one has gotten to know the target, there is much greater stability in the relationship effect. For instance, in the Park and Judd (1989) study, the day-to-day stability is .76. For Malloy (1987a), the correlation in the relationship effect from the middle to the end of the semester averages to .68. So there is not much stability in the relationship effect from zero acquaintance to initial interaction, but once the perceiver has an interaction history with the target, there is greater stability.

There is strong evidence that the relationship component changes at a faster rate than the target effect. As can be determined from Table 4.5 in Chapter 4, the stability of the target effect for Extroversion after zero acquaintance averages to .79, which is much greater than the .27 stability for the relationship effect. In addition, the Park and Judd (1989) study shows that the stability of the relationship effect is .76, whereas the day-to-day stability of the target effect in that study is about .98. Malloy (1987a) shows a similar pattern. Idiosyncratic impressions seem to be more variable than are consensual impressions. Perhaps the old saying that "First impressions are lasting impressions" needs to be modified: "Consensual first impressions, but not idiosyncratic first impressions, are lasting impressions." The relatively changeable nature of relationship suggests that mood or another very transitory factor is in part responsible for uniqueness.

Summary

Because in many studies uniqueness represents the largest source of variance, it deserves far greater attention in the study of interpersonal perception than it has received in the past. Compared to consensus, not very much is known about uniqueness. It is relatively easier for researchers to think about social perception as fundamentally a process that is individually based. Schemas, biases, and accuracy in interpersonal perception are relatively easy to understand, but it is more difficult to understand the relational aspect. The study of relationships is a science in its infancy.

One possible explanation of relationship effects in interpersonal perception is that perceptions are closely tied to affect. This explanation has considerable validity. Moreover, as the perceiver and target become better acquainted, affect becomes increasingly correlated with other-perception.

Perhaps the most promising avenue of explanation is to examine the different meaning systems of perceivers. It may be that perceivers use fundamentally different rules to combine information in interpersonal perception. However, there currently exists little or no research on these important issues.

In the next chapter, the investigation of the relationship effect in interpersonal perception proceeds. The topic of Chapter 6 is reciprocity, or the matching of people's perceptions of each other. It is the first topic in this book that truly captures the interpersonal nature of person perception.

Notes

1. In the section on different meaning systems, affect is also discussed. There, affect that is based on target information leads to a different meaning or interpretation of behavior. In this section, affect *by itself* without any behavioral information leads to different trait judgments.

2. For a multiplicative model of the form $Y = a + bZ$, the model is additive after transformation when a constant (i.e., a) is subtracted from Y. Thus, the standard logarithmic transformation assumes that the intercept is at the origin (i.e., the level of measurement is at the ratio level).

3. Even if perceivers were using a combination of cues and not just a single cue, the model may still apply. What is crucial in the multiple-cue, equal-weight model is that all perceivers in one group use one set of rules, and all perceivers in the other group use a different set of rules.

Chapter 6

RECIPROCITY AND ASSUMED RECIPROCITY

If Zelda sees Heidi as intelligent, does Heidi see Zelda as intelligent? Do people see each other as mirror images? In regard to affect, if Zelda likes Heidi, does Heidi like Zelda? The question of reciprocity in social perception is fundamental. Markus and Zajonc (1985), in their review of cognitive theories in social psychology, stated the following: "The properties of social perception and social cognition that make them distinct are reciprocity and intersubjectivity" (p. 213). Reciprocity is the first question discussed in this book that requires that perception be two-sided—in other words, that each person be both perceiver and target.

Within the Social Relations Model (SRM), reciprocity can be separated into reciprocity at the individual level and reciprocity at the dyadic level. At the individual level, the reciprocity is called "generalized." The question is whether people who are seen by others as possessing a given trait also see others as possessing that same trait. At the dyadic level, the question conforms more closely to the usual reciprocity question: If Alice uniquely sees Betty as very intelligent, then does Betty uniquely see Alice as intelligent? In this chapter, reciprocity of trait judgments and affect is considered. Also considered in this chapter is the question of assumed reciprocity: If Joan likes Helen, does she think that Helen will like her? The chapter begins with a discussion of reciprocity of liking judgments, because, as will be seen, reciprocity is much greater for liking than it is for other-perception.

Parts of this chapter are adapted from Kenny and DePaulo (1993). Copyright 1993 by the American Psychological Association. Adapted by permission.

Reciprocity of Liking Judgments

Reciprocity of attraction is a cultural truism. Gouldner (1960) even speculated that there may be a universal human norm of reciprocity. Berscheid and Walster (1978) organized their book on attraction by discussing exceptions to the general principle of reciprocity. Reciprocity seems obvious to both laypersons and social scientists.

It came as quite a surprise that early studies of attraction revealed little or no reciprocity. Evidence was so dismal that in 1979 Theodore Newcomb, then the dean of attraction researchers, published an article entitled "Reciprocity of Interpersonal Attraction: A Nonconfirmation of a Plausible Hypothesis."

As a graduate student in the early 1970s, I can remember my disappointment in analyzing a data set in which I found little or no evidence of reciprocity. It was this disappointment that in part led to the development of SRM. Once that model was developed, reciprocity of attraction was the first question that my colleagues and I investigated (Kenny & La Voie, 1982, 1984; Kenny & Nasby, 1980).

Table 6.1 (adapted from Table 3 of Kenny, 1994) presents the generalized- and dyadic-reciprocity correlations from several studies. The generalized-reciprocity correlation assesses the extent to which people who are liked by others (i.e., popular people) tend to like other people. The results in Table 6.1 for this type of reciprocity present an inconsistent pattern: Some generalized-reciprocity correlations are positive and others are negative. Two of these correlations have not even been computed because there is insufficient variance (less than 10%) in either the perceiver or the target effect. The average of the generalized-reciprocity correlations that are computed is only .19.

There is an explanation for why generalized reciprocity is virtually zero. We (Kenny & Nasby, 1980) speculated that there are two processes that bring about the perceiver–target correlation for liking. First, there is evidence that likers are liked (Folkes & Sears, 1977): People who like others may tend to be liked back. Second, there may be a negative causal path from the target effect to the perceiver effect. If people are liked by others, they can afford to be more choosy about whom they like. Given that the average perceiver–target correlation is near zero, it would appear that these two tendencies cancel out each other.

For dyadic reciprocity, the picture is quite different. In Table 6.1, all the dyadic correlations are based on multiple replications, and so error variance has been removed. There is quite impressive evidence of dyadic reciprocity. If Art likes Bob especially, then Bob especially likes Art. The results in Table 6.1 also clearly reveal that dyadic

TABLE 6.1. Reciprocity Correlations for Liking at the Generalized and Dyadic Levels

Study	Generalized	Dyadic
First encounters: One-on-one		
Burleson (1983)	.27	.26
Chapdelaine, Kenny, & LaFontana (in press)	.58	.42
Kenny & Bernstein (1982)	##	.29
First encounters: Groups		
Dabbs & Ruback (1987)	.36	.13
Kashy (1988)	.09	.28
Park & Flink (1989)	−.10	.18
Long-term acquaintance		
Burleson (1983)	.12	.49
Curry & Emerson (1970)	−.26	.48
Malloy & Albright (1990)	##	.75
Newcomb (1961)	—[a]	.58
Wright, Ingraham, & Blackmer (1985)	.49	.74

Note. ## insufficient variance to compute the correlation. Adapted from Kenny (1994).
Copyright 1994 by Lawrence Erlbaum Associates, Inc. Adapted by permission.
[a]Because ranks were used, perceiver variance cannot be computed.

reciprocity tends to increase with acquaintance. The average reciprocity correlation in the short-term acquaintance studies is .26, and rises to .61 in the long-term acquaintance studies. So, from short- to long-term acquaintance, the dyadic-reciprocity correlation more than doubles.

The results in Table 6.1 make clear why researchers who did not use SRM had difficulty finding reciprocity of attraction. The simple correlation of how much Alice likes Betty and how much Betty likes Alice contains a mix of the generalized and dyadic correlations (Kenny & Nasby, 1980). Because the generalized correlations are so small, they dilute the level of reciprocity in dyadic relations.

Although for some 10 years it has been known that reciprocity of liking increases with greater acquaintance, there is not a commonly accepted explanation of why such an increase exists. There are at least four possible explanations.

Traditionally in social psychology, the dominant theoretical explanation of interpersonal attraction has been "exchange theory." In exchange theory, the liking of another is presumed to be determined by the rewards that a person obtains from the interaction. So the reason John likes Marsha is based on the rewards that he receives when he is with Marsha. The definition of rewards is never clear in exchange theory.

If liking is determined by the rewards obtained in the interaction, to explain reciprocity of liking it must be assumed that the rewards of interaction are reciprocal: If Alice feels rewarded in interacting with Betty, then Betty also feels rewarded. If rewards are reciprocal (which seems plausible), if liking depends on the sheer number of rewards received in the relationship, and if relationships increasingly differ in the rewards received, then it would follow that there should be increases in reciprocity over time. Because it is difficult to measure rewards in interaction, this explanation of increasing reciprocity is not easily tested.

Another explanation of the increased reciprocity can be taken from Bem's (1967) self-perception theory. When people try to decide how much they like someone, they examine their own behavior to determine their liking. The cue that they use to infer their liking is frequency of interaction. Because frequency is itself reciprocal (i.e., the more time that Alice is with Betty, the more time Betty is with Alice), then liking must be reciprocal if dyads differ in the amount of interaction. It must also be assumed that people know how much time they spend with others—something that they appear to know (see Kashy & Kenny, 1990a, which is discussed in Chapter 7). So if people infer their liking from the cue of frequency of interaction, then liking should be reciprocal.

It is important to realize not only that acquaintance leads to attraction, but also that attraction leads to acquaintance. Normally, people wish to spend time with those they like. So a correlation between acquaintance and liking does not necessarily mean that acquaintance caused liking.

The third explanation of reciprocity is based on meta-perception. First, as is explained later in this chapter, there is strong evidence for assumed reciprocity: If Jack likes Jill, Jack presumes that Jill likes him. Assumed-reciprocity correlations are some of the largest correlations in interpersonal perception. Second, this explanation assumes that people's meta-perceptions of liking become increasingly accurate over time; that is, people know how others see them. The combination of assumed reciprocity and meta-accuracy results in reciprocity. Basically, how much Alice likes Betty causes Betty's meta-perception of how much Alice likes Betty, and then this meta-perception determines how much Betty likes Alice. I know of no actual evidence that dyadic meta-accuracy increases with acquaintance. But if it does, the combination of assumed reciprocity and meta-accuracy necessarily leads to increased reciprocity. So reciprocity is a by-product of meta-accuracy and assumed reciprocity.

The final explanation focuses on the effects of similarity on attraction. If actual similarity in attitudes, background, and values determines attraction, and if it takes time for this effect to emerge, there should be increasing reciprocity with increasing acquaintance. Byrne (1971) has considered the effects of similarity on attraction in great detail.

Which of these four explanations explains the increase in reciprocity as a function of acquaintance? It is likely that each plays a role, but currently the relative contribution of the four is unknown.

Reciprocity of Trait Judgments: Generalized Reciprocity

The question in this section is the correlation between a person's perceiver and target effects. For example, if John is seen by his peers as intelligent, does John in turn see his peers as intelligent? Historically, the correlation between the perceiver effect and the target effect has been interpreted as a measure of projection. "Projection," a psychoanalytic concept, means that people see traits in others that they *deny* that they have. In projection, it is assumed that the actual standing causes the perceiver effect for some people. For instance, a person may believe that he or she has a homosexual orientation, but this belief creates so much anxiety and guilt that he or she "projects" this orientation onto others, while simultaneously denying that he or she is homosexual. Thus, classical psychoanalytic projection does not necessarily imply a correlation between the perceiver and target effects.[1]

There are three fundamentally different processes that can result in a linkage between perceiver and target effects: self-perception, complementary projection, and misattribution. Interestingly, all three of these explanations presume that the target effect accurately reflects the person's behavior—in other words, that there is target accuracy (see Chapter 7). These three different theories are discussed, and then the research evidence concerning a perceiver–target correlation is reviewed.

Self-Perception

The topic in Chapter 9 is assumed similarity: Do people see others as they see themselves? If it is assumed that others see the persons as they view themselves (i.e., self–other agreement), then the combination of assumed similarity and self–other agreement implies that the perceiver and target effects are correlated. So if John thinks that he is stupid and so do other people, and if John thinks that others are like him (i.e., they are stupid), then there should be a correlation between the perceiver and target effects: John is seen by others as stupid, and he thinks that others are stupid.

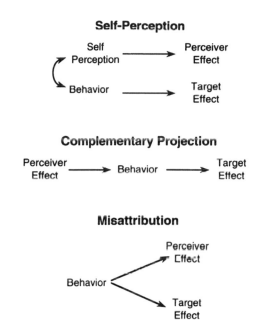

FIGURE 6.1. Three models that imply a perceiver–target correlation.

This pattern is illustrated in the top panel of Figure 6.1. A person's self-concept causes the person's perceiver effect. The self-concept is correlated with the person's behavior, and the behavior causes the target effect.

Generally, it is assumed that a person sees others as he or she sees himself or herself. People assume that others are like them, not different from them. Alternatively, there could be "assumed dissimilarity" or what has been called "contrast projection" (Campbell, Miller, Lubetsky, & O'Connell, 1964): People see others as different from themselves. For instance, if a person is not very intelligent, then that person may see others as very intelligent because he or she compares others to himself or herself. So, as discussed in Chapter 3, the self is used to anchor the scale, and people rate others in relation to themselves. Thus, if a person sees himself or herself the way others see him or her (there is self-other agreement), and if a person compares others to himself or herself (i.e., the self is used as a standard to judge others), then there should be negative perceiver–target correlations. According to Campbell et al. (1964), there is weak but consistent evidence supporting contrast projection. However, I have questioned this conclusion on statistical grounds (Kenny, 1981). Evidence about contrast and similarity projection is reviewed later in this chapter.

Complementary Projection

In "complementary projection" people may adopt various person-alities to fit into a world that they perceive. So if a person sees others as hostile, he or she may well adopt a hostile personality. Complementary projection predicts assumed similarity for some traits (Agreeableness) and contrast for other traits (Extroversion). For still other traits, it predicts that a perceiver effect for one trait implies a target effect for another trait. So, for example, if a person thinks that others are incompetent, he or she will be bossy in his or her interactions. In complementary projection, the direction of causation is from the perceiver effect to the target effect: A person's view of others changes how he or she behaves, and in turn changes others' perceptions of him or her. Note that it is assumed that behavior leads to accurate perception (target accuracy).

The model assumed by complementary projection is presented in the middle panel of Figure 6.1. The perceiver effect causes the person's behavior, and that behavior in turn causes the target effect.

Campbell et al. (1964) also discussed the possibility that the target effect may cause the perceiver effect in a form of complementary projection. For example, people may view a certain person as hostile (a target effect). This person (the perceiver) may rationalize his or her hostile actions because he or she thinks that others are hostile. So the perceiver effect serves as a rationalization or an excuse for this person's behavior. Again, the person's view of others complements his or her personality; however, in this case the causation goes from the person's behavior, which is indexed by the target effect, to the perceiver effect.

Misattribution

It is a truism that a person's behavior affects the behavior of his or her interaction partner. If a person is friendly, the people with whom that person interacts will probably behave in a friendly fashion. Given that the target is veridically perceived (people who are seen as friendly behave in a friendly manner), then friendly people should tend to have friendly interaction partners. If people fail to realize the effect of their behavior on others, which is something they seem to do (Gilbert & Jones, 1986), then there should be a perceiver effect to match the target effect. Campbell et al. (1964) referred to this phenomenon as "reactivity"; I prefer to use the more contemporary term of "misattribution." People fail to realize that they, not their partners, are the cause of their partners' behavior.

In the bottom panel of Figure 6.1, the misattribution model is presented. A person's behavior causes both the target and perceiver effect. It is interesting to note that all three models illustrated in Figure 6.1 presume target accuracy: A person's behavior causes his or her target effect.

Empirical Results

What is the correlation between the perceiver and target effects? Table 6.2 presents the perceiver–target correlations from 12 different studies. For each study I have computed the median perceiver–target correlation. The average perceiver–target correlation is a paltry − .01. There is then not much evidence for a correlation between perceiver and target effects.

An overall zero correlation could be a result of negative and positive correlations canceling each other out. To investigate this possibility, I have examined the perceiver–target correlations from the Park and Judd (1989) study. In that study there was no interaction, and people merely asked each other a standard set of questions. So in this study, the perceiver–target correlation could not reflect misattribution because

TABLE 6.2. Generalized and Dyadic Reciprocity Correlations of Trait Judgments

Study	Generalized	Dyadic
Short-term acquaintance: One-on-one		
Chapdelaine et al. (in press)	.18	.06
Reno & Kenny (1992)	.04	.01
Oliver (1989)	.16	.10
Short-term acquaintance: group		
Levesque (1990)	− .08	.04
Rothbart & Singer (1988)	.12	− .02
Hallmark & Kenny (1989)	− .00	− .01
Kashy (1988)	− .12	− .03
Shechtman & Kenny (in press)	.00	.04
Long-term acquaintance		
Dantchik (1985)	− .11	.01
Malloy & Albright (1990)	− .28	.16
Albright, Kenny, & Malloy (1988) Study 1	− .02	.03
Campbell, Miller, Lubetsky, & O'Connell (1964)	.04	.11
Mean	− .01	.04

the two people did not interact with each other in the usual sense. Thus, the resulting perceiver–target correlation must be attributable to either complementary projection, assumed similarity, or contrast projection. I have divided the traits into the Big Five factors and computed the median perceiver–target correlation.

Table 6.3 presents the results from this analysis. As seen in the table, there is evidence for a positive perceiver–target correlation for Agreeableness and negative correlations for Extroversion and Culture. What is the explanation for this pattern of results? The pattern is certainly not supportive of assumed similarity, in that for two of the five factors the correlation is negative. Though somewhat supportive of contrast projection, the positive correlation for Agreeableness undermines that explanation. Complementary projection would predict the positive correlation for Agreeableness, and the negative correlations for Extroversion and Culture are somewhat consistent with complementary projection. So there is some support for complementary projection.

It should be realized that the correlations in Table 6.3 are rather small. Because all the models that attempt to explain the perceiver–target correlation presume that there is correspondence between how a person behaves and others' perceptions of that person, no doubt that correspondence is far from perfect. That is, low to moderate target accuracy probably greatly diminishes the magnitude of the perceiver–target correlation.

There is a test for misattribution through an examination of one-on-one interactions with strangers. If Alice tends to behave in a friendly way, and Alice makes her partners also behave in that way, then perhaps Alice will see her partners as also friendly. Table 6.4 presents the perceiver–target correlations from two one-on-one studies. Table 6.4 does provide evidence that there is misattribution for the factor Agreeableness. Note that it has the most positive correlation in both studies. Of course, the correlation for Agreeableness could be a resultl of other processes besides misattribution.

TABLE 6.3. Median Generalized-Reciprocity Correlations Based on Data from the Park and Judd (1989) Study

Factor	Number of traits	Correlation
Extroversion	18	− .12
Agreeableness	16	.15
Conscientiousness	8	− .00
Emotional Stability	8	.03
Culture	4	− .19

TABLE 6.4. Median Generalized-Reciprocity Correlations from
Two One-on-One Studies

Factor	Chapdelaine et al. (in press)	Reno & Kenny (1992)
Extroversion	.09	.15
Agreeableness	.19	.23
Conscientiousness	.03	−.48
Emotional Stability	.14	.03
Culture	.11	−.22

Overall, there is very little evidence for a perceiver–target correlation. There is some weak evidence for complementary projection in
the Park and Judd (1989) study, and there is evidence for misattribution of Agreeableness in two one-on-one studies. The one consistent
result is a correlation for Agreeableness.

Reciprocity of Trait Perception: Dyadic Reciprocity

The question of dyadic reciprocity of traits is as follows: If John sees
Henry as particularly intelligent, does Henry see John as particularly
intelligent? Why would there be any expectation of dyadic reciprocity
for traits? Considered here are two explanations of dyadic reciprocity
of other-perception, each of which relies on reciprocity at another level.
First, it is reasonable to believe that some behaviors are reciprocal (Cappella, 1981). Most likely, prosocial and antisocial behaviors are likely to be reciprocal. If I smile when I interact with you, you will probably
smile too. Simply put, if Alice is nice to Betty, then Betty is likely to
be nice to Alice. (Actually, research has provided stronger evidence
for the converse: If Alice is nasty to Betty, Betty is likely to be nasty
to Alice. See Kelley & Stahelski, 1970.) If there is reciprocity in behavior between interaction partners and if trait perception is tied to
behavior, then there should be some reciprocity in perceptions.
    Second, given that trait perceptions are at least in part driven by
affect, and given that there is reciprocity in affective judgments, then
there should be a reciprocity in trait judgments. Because it is known
that the correlation between affect and liking is about .65 (see Chapter 5, Table 5.1), and that, at least among well-acquainted people, the
level of dyadic reciprocity is about .6 (see Table 6.1), then statistically the expectation is for a correlation of about .4 (.65 × .6) for dyadic reciprocity for trait perception. If it is assumed that about one-half

of the relationship variance is error variance (see Table 5.1), then a good guess for the dyadic-reciprocity correlation would be about .20.

In Table 6.2 above, the dyadic-reciprocity correlations across 12 studies have been presented. As seen in the table, there is little or no evidence of reciprocity of perceptions in trait judgments, the average of the 12 correlations being only .04. If the focus is only on the well-acquainted dyads, there is a somewhat higher correlation of .08, but it is still much lower than the predicted correlation of .20.

What happens when the dyadic correlations are broken down by trait type? Because both the reciprocal-behavior theory and the liking theory imply a dyadic correlation for Agreeableness, that factor should evidence dyadic reciprocity. Table 6.5 presents the correlations from two one-on-one studies that should have large amounts of relationship variance. The results in the table show that there is very little reciprocity in trait perceptions. The only trait with a hint of a correlation is Extroversion, but that correlation is very small.[2]

The weak dyadic-reciprocity correlations of trait perceptions suggest that trait perception and affect are fairly independent: Affect is reciprocal and trait judgments are not. However, as Chapter 5 has clearly shown, affect and trait perceptions are strongly correlated. It is a puzzle that currently has no definitive solution. Consider the implications of the contradiction for the direction of the affect–cognition causal effects.

If the assumption is that affect causes trait judgments, there is the problem that there should be a more positive correlation between trait judgments. The only way to offset the correlation is to assume that the behavioral correlation is negative. Although negative correlations for Extroversion make some sense, it seems unlikely that the other factors have negative correlations.

Alternatively, if the correlation goes from trait judgment to affect, then it is necessary to supplement the reciprocity in affect. This is less problematic. It need only be assumed that once trait effects are

TABLE 6.5. Median Dyadic-Reciprocity Correlations from Two One-on-One Studies

Factor	Chapdelaine et al. (in press)	Reno & Kenny (1992)
Extroversion	.19	.08
Agreeableness	− .04	− .06
Conscientiousness	.01	− .04
Emotional Stability	.06	.07
Culture	.06	− .01

controlled, the dyadic-reciprocity correlation for affect is very large, approaching 1. Because this is more plausible than negative behavioral reciprocity, there is support for the idea that trait judgment causes affect more than affect causes trait judgment. Clearly, more research is needed to explore the linkages between trait judgments and affect.

Assumed Reciprocity

Perceivers realize that their targets are perceiving them. Consequently, people often engage in meta-perception: They try to perceive another person's perception of them. In this section, two different topics concerning the reciprocity of meta-perceptions are discussed. In the first, Jack attempts to perceive how others perceive him; in the second, Jack perceives how two different people see each other. In discussing these two topics, I rely on another analysis (Kenny & DePaulo, 1993) and a recent study (Chapdelaine, Kenny, & LaFontana, in press), respectively.

Meta-Perceptions of the Self

People may assume that there is reciprocity in people's liking for each other and in their evaluation of each other's traits. If Jack sees Jill as good-natured, he may simply assume that Jill will also see him as good-natured. He may do so without even bothering to look at Jill to see whether she seems to be regarding him as good-natured.

We (Kenny & DePaulo, 1993) analyzed eight studies to evaluate perceived and actual reciprocity in perception. To evaluate the assumed-reciprocity hypothesis, it must be determined whether people really do assume reciprocity and whether reciprocity does in fact exist. Table 6.6 presents the correlations for both the actual dyadic reciprocity of impressions (if Jack sees Jill as sociable, does Jill see Jack as sociable?) and the assumed reciprocity between meta-perception and the impression (if Jack sees Jill as sociable, does he think that Jill sees him as sociable?). When relationship and error variance can be separated because there are multiple measures, and there is sufficient relationship variance, the dyadic correlations can be adjusted to remove the effects of error. These correlations are presented in the last two columns of Table 6.6.

The top of Table 6.6 presents the correlations for actual and assumed reciprocities in trait studies. With hardly any exception, neither type of reciprocity is very strong. So if Jack sees Jill as good-natured

TABLE 6.6. Corrrelations for Dyadic Reciprocity, Actual and Assumed

Study	Unadjusted		Adjusted[a]	
	Actual	Assumed	Actual	Assumed
Trait				
Anderson (1985)	.14	.17	xx	xx
DePaulo, Kenny, Hoover, Webb, & Oliver (1987)	.12	.32	.25	.61
Kenny & DePaulo (1990)				
Applicant	− .01[b]	.09	##	##
Interviewer	− .01[b]	.12	##	##
Malloy & Albright (1990)	.11	.10	xx	xx
Malloy & Janowski (1992)	− .06	.10	− .08	.13
Oliver (1989)	.11	− .23	xx	xx
Reno & Kenny (1992)	.14	.42	xx	xx
Affect				
Curry & Emerson (1970)				
Week 1	.40	.61	xx	xx
Week 8	.53	.74	xx	xx
DePaulo et al. (1987)	.27	.70	.19	.82
Kenny & DePaulo (1990)				
Applicant	− .11[b]	.67	− .13[b]	##
Interviewer	− .11[b]	.46	− .13[b]	.59
Oliver (1989)	.35	.29	xx	xx
Reno & Kenny (1992)	.12	.47	xx	xx
Mean	.21	.56		

Note. ## = less than 5% of the variance; correlation not computed; xx = single replication, adjustment not possible. Adapted from Kenny and DePaulo (1993). Copyright 1993 by the American Psychological Association. Adapted by permission.
[a]Error removed from relationship effects.
[b]Actual reciprocity is the same for applicant and interviewer.

or intelligent, Jill will not necessarily see Jack in those ways. Furthermore, Jack does not necessarily assume that Jill sees his good-natured personality or his intelligence in the same way that he sees hers. For six of the eight comparisons, perceptions of reciprocity are stronger than actual reciprocity, but the levels of assumed reciprocity are not high.

The bottom of Table 6.6 presents the correlations for actual and assumed reciprocities in studies of affect. Both types of reciprocity are higher than the corresponding reciprocities for traits. Therefore, for affect, there is both actual reciprocity (if Jack likes Jill, Jill likes Jack) and assumed reciprocity (if Jack likes Jill, he thinks that Jill likes him). There may be more actual reciprocity for liking than there is for traits, because people are likely to feel positive toward someone who feels positive toward them; it is less likely that people will think someone else is witty just because that someone thinks they are witty.

In six of the seven comparisons, it can be seen that subjects assumed more reciprocity of liking—sometimes much more—than actually existed. Assumed reciprocity of liking is substantial for virtually every study; the median for the seven correlations is .61. Note that this correlation is not corrected for attenuation, and so if they were corrected, the correlations would be virtually 1.

It can also be asked to what extent people believe that if someone is popular, he or she will like others. At issue is the correlation between the target effect in liking and the target effect in meta-perception. It can also be asked whether those who tend to like others also tend to think that they are liked by others. This latter correlation is between the perceiver effects in other- and meta-perception. Table 6.7 presents these results.

Both sets of correlations are very impressive. The "smallest" correlation in the table is .69. Thus, there is strong evidence that assumed reciprocity operates at the individual level. Popular people are assumed to like others, and if a person likes others, this person assumes that others like him or her. Assumed reciprocity operates at both the individual and dyadic levels.

TABLE 6.7. Correlations for Assumed Reciprocity of Affect at the Individual Level

Study	Target	Perceiver
Curry & Emerson (1970)		
Week 1	.89	.76
Week 8	1.00	.90
DePaulo et al. (1987)	##	.83
Kenny & DePaulo (1990)		
Applicant	##	.98
Interviewer	##	.85
Oliver (1989)	##	##
Reno & Kenny (1992)	##	.69

Note. ## = less than 5% of the variance; correlation not computed.

Meta-Perceptions of Others

When people are asked to state how much other people like each other, these are perceptions of liking. These perceptions are similar to meta-perceptions of liking (just discussed); however, people are not asked how much somebody likes them, but rather how much somebody likes somebody else. The question is whether there is reciprocity of liking in these judgments. Just to be clear, the question concerns asking Zelda how much she thinks Heidi likes Carol.

We (Chapdelaine et al., in press) conducted a study to examine this question. We had groups of five women, who were initially strangers, interact one-on-one for 10 minutes per interaction. The women were told that they would later make predictions about one another. After each interaction, the two participants were encouraged to take notes, and each woman completed a form asking her how much she liked her interaction partner. After each woman had interacted with each of the four other women, she predicted how much the other four women would like one another. So each woman made a total of 12 predictions.

We computed individual- and dyadic-reciprocity coefficients for the predictions of each woman. We found reciprocity correlations at the individual level of .68. However, actual reciprocity at the individual level in this study was .58 (see Table 6.1). So people think that popular people like others more than they really do like others.

At the dyadic level, the assumed-reciprocity correlation was .53. When appropriate corrections were made to remove error variance, it was found that the dyadic-reciprocity correlation was essentially 1.00. Thus, people assume that if Art likes Bob, then Bob must like Art. The actual dyadic-reciprocity correlation was lower, being .42.

Frey and Smith (1993) conducted a similar study (see their Study 2). They had people predict how much their friends liked each other. They replicated the high level of reciprocity of perceived liking judgments that we (Chapdelaine et al., in press) found. Moreover, they found even higher levels of assumed generalized reciprocity, .85. They too found that people assumed that popular people liked others — an assumption that is generally false (see the first column of numbers in Table 6.1).

Summary

There appears to be no evidence of individual-level reciprocity of attraction: Popular people do not tend to like others any more than unpopular people. However, people seem to assume mistakenly that popular people do like others. At the dyadic level, there is strong evidence that when the two participants know each other well, there is reciprocity of attraction. Reciprocity of attraction, then, exists at the dyadic and not the individual level of analysis.

Overall, trait judgments do not show either individual or dyadic reciprocity. However, at the individual level, there is some weak evidence of individual-level reciprocity of Agreeableness: If a person sees others as agreeable, he or she is seen by others as agreeable. Dyadic-level correlations are consistently weak.

A continual undercurrent in the investigation of reciprocity of perception is the question of reciprocity of behavior. A systematic examination of evidence concerning reciprocity of behavior is needed. Particularly important is the extent to which both prosocial behavior and antisocial behavior are reciprocated.

People assume that if they like someone, that person likes them. They also assume that liking is reciprocal when they guess at how much people like one another. So assumed reciprocity of liking is the norm. There is no evidence for assumed reciprocity of traits.

This chapter, perhaps more than any other in the book, is filled with speculation. Despite the early initial interest in investigating reciprocity of attraction using SRM, there has been little recent investigation of the topic. This is unfortunate, and I hope that the future will result in renewed interest in this most interesting topic.

Notes

1. It should be pointed out that researchers often use the term "projection" when the person doing the projecting is aware of his or her standing on the trait. Because the term "projection" requires denial, these are not cases of projection as classically defined.

2. Extensive research shows that friends are more similar to one another than are nonfriends. This is not the same as dyadic reciprocity, but rather a correlation in target effects (Kenny & Kashy, in press).

TARGET ACCURACY

Accuracy in interpersonal perception is a fundamental issue in social and personality psychology. Are people's perceptions of others valid? This is the most obvious question in the field of interpersonal perception, yet, surprisingly, the most difficult to study.

Common sense suggests that people do have some idea about what other people are like. We all presume that we have some insight into the personalities of our lovers, parents, friends, and bosses. Some understanding of the social world seems necessary if an individual is to survive (Fiske, 1993; McArthur & Baron, 1983; Swann, 1984).[1]

The chapter begins with a historical review of the topic and of the Cronbach and Gage critique of global accuracy scores. On the basis of this review, it is concluded that accuracy research should be nomothetic, interpersonal, and componential; it is also shown how the Social Relations Model (SRM) fulfills these requirements and provides a methodology to study interpersonal accuracy. Next discussed is how the measurement of the criterion (what a person is really like) presents additional problems in accuracy research. Results from two accuracy studies are presented. Finally, the Weighted-Average Model (WAM), developed in Chapter 4, is applied to the question of target accuracy. The present chapter represents a substantial update of an earlier analysis (Kenny & Albright, 1987) of accuracy.

Historical Survey

Accuracy in person perception is one of the oldest topics in social and personality psychology. Its roots lie in the success of standardized in-

Parts of this chapter are adapted from Kenny (1986) and Kenny and Albright (1987). Copyright 1986 and 1987 by William D. Crano and the American Psychological Association, respectively. Adapted by permission.

telligence testing. Researchers reasoned that if it were possible to measure individual differences in cognitive skills, then it should be possible to measure individual differences in social skills. Psychologists rushed to the task of measuring individual differences in accuracy in person perception. Whether it was called "accuracy," "empathy," "social skills," "understanding" or "sensitivity," the goal was always essentially the same: to differentiate people by their ability to know the social world surrounding them.

The individual-difference orientation fostered during World War II in the United States easily absorbed this tradition. Social scientists were eager to select individuals who could be leaders and be responsive to the demands of the troops they commanded.

After World War II, the aims of accuracy researchers continued to focus on selection. But the emphasis shifted to the selection of clinicians, social workers, and teachers, who were thought to be skilled perceivers of people. Also, poorly adjusted people were thought to be those who were inaccurate person perceivers. In the late 1940s and early 1950s, the study of individual differences in the accuracy of social perception became a dominant area of research in social and personality psychology.

Critique of Accuracy Research

In the mid-1950s, all of the interest in and enthusiasm about accuracy research came to a crashing halt. Several prominent psychometricians, most notably Cronbach and Gage (Cronbach, 1955, 1958; Gage & Cronbach, 1955; Gage, Leavitt, & Stone, 1956), called into question the measurement techniques of the accuracy researchers. These researchers did not argue that accuracy could not be measured (as is sometimes mistakenly thought), but that a complete treatment of accuracy required much more complicated procedures than those available then. Because these criticisms are so important and are not well understood, I review them here in detail. I also show that the approach taken in this chapter parallels the Cronbach (1955) components.

Cronbach (1955) distinguished among four components of accuracy: "elevation," "differential elevation," "stereotype accuracy," and "differential accuracy."[2] To understand these terms, a detailed consideration of the judgment process is required.

Each perceiver rates a set of targets on a set of traits. For each judgment, there is a criterion score, the target's actual standing on the trait. (This chapter later considers the measurement of the criterion.) "Accuracy" is generally defined as the correspondence between the judgment and the criterion (Kruglanski, 1989). Often the measure of accuracy is the average of the discrepancies between the judgments and the criterion. Cronbach (1955) criticized the use of a single, global discrepancy score as a measure of accuracy. The reasons for his reservations about such measures are now explained.

Partitioning Judgments

I review an earlier presentation here (Kenny, 1986). Consider the ratings of a particular judge of a set of targets on a set of traits, as in Table 7.1a. There are three targets (Mary, Jane, and Beth) and three traits ("intelligent," "friendly," and "honest"). It is assumed that the judge, who will be called Sandy, has rated the three targets on a 10-point scale for each trait. (For the moment, ignore Table 7.1b.)

Table 7.2a presents the criterion scores for the same three targets and the same three traits. It is assumed that the targets obtained these scores on three highly reliable, standardized tests of intelligence, friendliness, and honesty. The criterion measures, like the judgments, range from 1 to 10. Scores are oriented so that higher scores indicate more favorable ratings. It is the correspondence between Sandy's judgments

TABLE 7.1. Judgments and Partitioning of Judgments about Three Targets on Three Traits

a. *Judgments*

Traits	Targets		
	Mary	Jane	Beth
Intelligent	10	7	4
Friendly	6	8	1
Honest	2	3	4

b. *Partitioned Judgments*

Traits	Targets			Trait effect scores
	Mary	Jane	Beth	
Intelligent	2	−1	−1	2
Friendly	0	2	−2	0
Honest	−2	−1	3	−2
Target effect scores	1	1	−2	5[a]

Note. Uniqueness scores are boxed in. Adapted from Kenny (1986). Copyright 1986 by William D. Crano. Adapted by permission.
[a]Constant score for judge.

TABLE 7.2. Criterion Scores and Partitioned Criterion Scores of Three Targets on Three Traits

a. *Criterion Scores*

Traits	Targets		
	Mary	Jane	Beth
Intelligent	7	8	9
Friendly	7	4	7
Honest	1	3	8

b. *Partitioned Criterion Scores*

Traits	Targets			Trait effect scores
	Mary	Jane	Beth	
Intelligent	0	1	−1	2
Friendly	2	1	1	0
Honest	−2	0	2	−2
Target effect scores	−1	−1	2	6[a]

Note. Uniqueness scores are boxed in. Adapted from Kenny (1986). Copyright 1986 by William D. Crano. Adapted by permission.
[a]Constant score for criterion.

(Table 7.1a) and the criterion scores (Table 7.2a) that is at issue in the consideration of interpersonal accuracy.

The judgments and the criterion scores can each be divided into component parts. As seen later in the chapter, the relationships between these parts define Cronbach's four types of accuracy. In Table 7.1b, Sandy's judgments have been divided into four components. In equation form, this partitioning is as follows:

Judgment = Constant + Trait + Target + Uniqueness

(This decomposition can be viewed as a two-way analysis of variance, in which trait and target are main effects and uniqueness is the interaction between the two.)

Consider Sandy's judgment that Mary scores a 10 in intelligence. According to the formula, the 10 is the total of the constant term plus the trait term plus the target term plus the uniqueness term. These four components and their derivation are described in the following paragraphs.

The "constant term" is the tendency for the judge to rate *all* the targets on *all* the traits either favorably or unfavorably. It represents a very general response set, because it affects the judgments of every target on every trait. The constant is the average of all of Sandy's nine judgments, as presented in Table 7.1a. Thus, Sandy's constant score is $+5$, and this is indicated in the bottom right-hand corner of Table 7.1b. Because the ratings can range from 1 to 10, with 5.5 as the scale midpoint, a score of 5 indicates that Sandy is relatively neutral in her overall rating of the targets.

The "trait effect" represents the judge's tendency to view a particular trait as being high or low *relative to the other traits that are rated*. The trait effect is the average of Sandy's judgments for a specific trait minus the constant effect. So for intelligence, the trait effect is $(10 + 7 + 4)/3 - 5$, which equals 2. The trait effect is specific to the trait that is being rated. Thus, for friendliness, the trait effect is $(6 + 8 + 1)/3 - 5$, or 0. Judgmental trait effects are noted in the final column of Table 7.1b. The entries in this column indicate that Sandy sees the targets as being relatively more intelligent than honest. Trait effects necessarily sum to zero.

The "target effect" (which is *not* the same as the target effect in SRM) represents any tendency for the judge to view a specific target more or less favorably than the other targets. It is computed in a manner parallel to that of the trait effect, except that the judgments are averaged for a particular target rather than for a trait. Thus, the target effect for Mary is $(10 + 6 + 2)/3 - 5$, which equals 1. Target effect scores are given in the bottom row of Table 7.1b, and they are 1 for Mary, as noted, 1 for Jane, and -2 for Beth. They, too, necessarily sum to zero. The hypothetical judge, Sandy, views Mary and Jane more favorably than she does Beth. The target effect may well represent how much the judge particularly likes the target.

The final component of the judgment score is what is called "uniqueness," which represents the judge's views of the target on a particular trait after the constant, the trait effect, and the target effect are removed. Basically, this measure indicates how the target is uniquely evaluated on the particular trait by the judge. The uniqueness score is computed by subtraction. It equals the judgment minus the constant, the trait, and the target effects. So for Sandy's judgment of Mary on the trait intelligent, the uniqueness component is $10 - 5 - 2 - 1$, which equals 2. The uniqueness scores are the boxed-in entries of Table 7.1b. They necessarily sum to zero across each target and across each trait.

The uniqueness component can provide information that appears somewhat at odds with the judgment data. Take, for example, Sandy's seemingly low rating of Beth on the trait of honesty. The uniqueness score for this rating is 3, which is the highest uniqueness score in Table

7.lb. The relatively large uniqueness score tells us that the low score of 4 is not really that low, because the target (Beth) tends to be rated low by Sandy on all measured traits. As such, for this judge's rating of this target on this trait, a 4 is a rather high rating.

Partitioning Criterion Scores and Defining Accuracy

In Table 7.2b, the criterion measure has been divided into the same components as the judgments. In equation form, the partitioning is as follows:

$$\text{Criterion} = \text{Constant} + \text{Trait} + \text{Target} + \text{Uniqueness}$$

The constant term is the average score on the criterion for all the targets on all the traits. The constant for the criterion is 6, 1 unit higher than Sandy's judgment constant. The trait effect represents any tendency for the targets to have more or less of the quantity being studied. So in this case, the three targets tend to be more intelligent than friendly, and more friendly than honest. The target effect represents any tendency for the targets to be high or low on the criterion. The target effects in the bottom row of Table 7.2b indicate that Beth scores higher on the traits than either Mary or Jane does. Finally, the last part of the criterion is uniqueness. This quantity represents the part in the criterion score for a given individual, on a specific trait, that remains after the constant, trait, and target effects are removed.

At last, Cronbach's (1955) four components can be discussed. Recall that Cronbach asserted that the simple average of the discrepancies between judgment and criterion for a judge consists of four different components. These components are diagrammed in Figure 7.1. At the top of Figure 7.1, the judgment is divided into four parts—constant, trait, target, and uniqueness. At the bottom of the figure, the criterion score is divided into the same four components. Cronbach's four components of accuracy can be viewed as linking together the corresponding parts of the judgment and the criterion scores.

"Elevation" concerns the degree of correspondence between the constant of the judgment and the constant of the criterion; that is, it is the discrepancy between the judge's average score and the average score that targets obtain on the criterion. Table 7.1b shows that Sandy, the judge, has an average score (or constant) of 5 over all the judgments made, and the average score (or constant) of the nine criterion scores in Table 7.2b is 6. As such, the elevation, or the discrepancy in constants, is only 1 unit on a 10-point scale.

"Stereotype accuracy" concerns the degree of correspondence

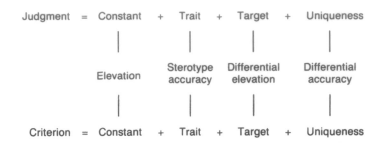

FIGURE 7.1. Cronbach's four components of accuracy. Adapted from Kenny and Albright (1987). Copyright 1987 by the American Psychological Association. Adapted by permission.

between the trait effects of the judgment and the trait effects of the criterion. This component of accuracy concerns whether the pattern of the average ratings of the traits of a judge corresponds to the pattern of the average score for the traits on the criterion. An examination of Tables 7.1b and 7.2b shows that there is an exact correspondence between the trait effects, which are presented in the last column of each of these tables. The trait effect is 2 for "intelligent," 0 for "friendly," and −2 for "honest" for both the judgment and the criterion.

"Differential elevation" involves the degree of correspondence between the target effects. This component of accuracy concerns whether the pattern of a judge's average ratings of the targets corresponds to the pattern of the average score for the targets on the criterion. Examination of Tables 7.1b and 7.2b reveals a perfect inverse relationship between the target effects, presented in the bottom rows of these two tables. The target effects for the judgments are 1 for Mary, 1 for Jane, and −2 for Beth, whereas the target effects for the criterion are −1 for Mary, −1 for Jane, and +2 for Beth.

"Differential accuracy" concerns the correspondence between corresponding uniqueness components. One way to measure differential accuracy is to correlate the uniqueness scores of the judgments with the uniqueness scores of the criterion.[3] So the pairs of scores would be correlated from the boxed-in sections of Tables 7.1b and 7.2b. Table 7.3 presents the two sets of uniqueness scores. The correlation between these variables is .47, which indicates that the judgments (after the removal of trait and target effects) agree with the criterion scores after the trait and target effects of the criterion measures have also been removed.

To summarize, the total accuracy score is partitioned into four

TABLE 7.3. Uniqueness Scores for Data from Tables 7.1 and 7.2

Judgment	Criterion
2	0
−1	1
−1	−1
0	2
2	0
−2	−1
−2	−2
−1	0
3	2

Note. Adapted from Kenny (1986). Copyright 1986 by William D. Crano. Adapted by permission.

components: elevation, stereotype accuracy, differential elevation, and differential accuracy. For the example in Tables 7.1 and 7.2, the elevation shows close correspondence between the constants; the stereotype accuracy shows perfect correspondence between the trait effects; the differential elevation shows an inverse correspondence between the target effects; and the differential accuracy shows moderate correspondence between the uniqueness scores.

According to Cronbach and others, only two of the four components that have been defined reflect meaningful accuracy: differential elevation and differential accuracy. The remaining components — elevation and stereotype accuracy[4] — involve the match between the judge's response set and the criterion.

If multiple targets and traits are used, the reliability of these components of accuracy can be assessed. Generally, it is difficult to measure differential accuracy, a component of true accuracy, reliably (see later section on nomothetic orientation). Particular care must be taken in interpreting the low reliability for differential accuracy. Low reliability in differential accuracy means that there are not *consistent* individual differences in differential accuracy. However, low reliability says nothing concerning whether, on average, persons score above chance levels in differential accuracy. Performance above chance levels can be tested by comparing the average differential accuracy to the level that would be expected if subjects were only guessing. If differential accuracy is measured by a correlation coefficient, then chance differential accuracy is a correlation of zero.

Postcritique Accuracy Research

Although the effect was unintended, Cronbach's accuracy critique stigmatized accuracy research. It became an unresearchable topic. No one wanted to investigate an area that was, according to Cline (1964), a "Pandora's box of 'components, artifacts, and methodological problems' (Cronbach, 1955)" (p. 227). A few brave souls continued to work on the topic, but it is fair to say that accuracy as an area of study withered away, and students were advised that it was a dead topic. Cook (1979) characterized the reaction as follows:

> The whole business of trying to measure the accuracy of person perception is so hopelessly complicated that it should be abandoned. This was the impression created on many researchers by Cronbach's critiques; the apparent difficulty of doing research led many workers in the field, by a familiar rationalization, to argue that the issue wasn't important, wasn't worth studying experimentally or even that it didn't exist. (p. 118)

Accuracy research "lost . . . its charm" (Schneider, Hastorf, & Ellsworth, 1979, p. 222).

What was to replace accuracy as an area of research? These criticisms extended beyond accuracy to any measure that was dyadic. Clearly, individual topics were safer and less subject to the rapier-like criticisms of such methodological experts as Cronbach. The field turned to attitudes in general and dissonance theory in particular. The current fascination with intrapsychic, cognitive topics in social psychology is a result, in part, of the Cronbach–Gage critique.

Research in person perception continued. Gage and Cronbach (1955) correctly predicted the dominant theme of research in person perception:

> Social perception as measured is a process dominated far more by what the Perceiver brings to it than by what he takes in during it. His favorability toward the Other, before or after he observes the Other, and his implicit personality theory, formed by his experiences prior to his interaction with the Other, seem to determine his perceptions. (p. 420)

No doubt, too, the "new look in perception" in the 1950s encouraged the field of person perception to move away from the study of accuracy to the study of bias. Subsequent work in person perception that carefully documents the human observer's use of heuristics, implicit assumptions, and egocentric orientation got its impetus from the end of accuracy research.

Even if one were willing to do Cronbach (1955) analyses, the com-

putational burden in that precomputer era was excessive. Most researchers already viewed the pre-Cronbach-and-Gage procedures available
at the time as complicated enough. The suggested added complexity
was too much. Various computations could not be done "because the
amount of calculation involved in obtaining them is prohibitive" (Cline
& Richards, 1960, p. 5). The results of all these computations were
very disappointing, and Cook (1979) drew the conclusion that "more
refined methods show that perceptions of other people are for the most
part very inaccurate" (p. 145).

Resurgence of Accuracy Research

The extensive literature on bias (cf. Higgins, Herman, & Zanna, 1981;
Nisbett & Ross, 1980), and the paucity of accuracy research, have
given social science a misleading picture of the person perceiver (Funder,
1987). It is known that observers make errors, but mistakes mean only
that person perceivers are not perfect. Even an expert tennis player
occasionally double-faults, makes unforced errors, and allows his or
her opponent to make passing shots. Very good batters in baseball
are out two-thirds of the time. Excellence and perfection are not syn-
onymous. Hastie and Rasinski (1988) showed that even though human
observers make mistakes, their accuracy can be quite high. Most tests
of bias take as the null hypothesis that people are totally accurate, and
show, not surprisingly, that indeed they are not perfectly accurate. To
determine the level of accuracy, one must measure it directly and not
infer it from a measure of bias.

Others besides Hastie and Rasinski (1988) have argued that person perceivers may be more accurate than one might think. McArthur
and Baron (1983) have taken an ecological approach. In part, they
have argued that an experimental context with verbal stimuli is not
representative of the typical human judgment situation. Swann (1984)
has said that accuracy lies not in judging people in general, but in judging specific interaction partners.

The Second Wave of Accuracy Research

If investigators want to see a rebirth of accuracy research, they must
take into account the complexities raised in the 1950s. In the hurry
to study accuracy, they must not repeat the mistakes of the past. Therefore, modern work on accuracy — the second wave — must be responsive to critiques of research from the 1950s. Our earlier analysis (Kenny

& Albright, 1987) has made it clear that accuracy research must be nomothetic, interpersonal, and componential.

Nomothetic Orientation

Most of the previous research in accuracy was in the area of individual differences. Recall that intelligence testing was the initial impetus for accuracy research. Both during World War II and in the postwar era, accuracy research had an avowed purpose: to select either the very able or the very unable.

Several converging sources of evidence point to small amounts of individual differences in accuracy. First, researchers following Cronbach and Gage have measured the reliability of differential accuracy. Their general finding is that reliability in this component is low. (Normally, .70 is considered minimally acceptable reliability.) Cronbach (1955) reported the reliability of differential accuracy as .18. Crow and Hammond (1957, Study 2) obtained over-time reliabilities in the .25 range for their measure of differential accuracy. Also, Bronfenbrenner, Harding, and Gallwey (1958) found reliability for this component to be nil (p. 52). These low reliabilities are not just true for older studies. In a more recent study, Anderson (1985) found an average reliability of .18 for differential accuracy across four traits. Cronbach's doubts in 1955 about "whether accuracy in differentiating personalities of others can be reliably measured" (p. 185) appear to be borne out.[5]

These low reliabilities can give a mistaken notion about validity. Measures of reliability assess the consistency of individual differences. If the reliability is low, it does not necessarily indicate that the average level of response is meaningless. A test can have no reliability, yet the mean or the average score can be interpretable. Imagine the following test of visual acuity in a classroom. An instructor writes a word on the blackboard and asks the students to copy it. The instructor does this 10 times. One can create a score from 0 to 10 to measure acuity. Presumably, most students would get 10's, but for various reasons there may be a few scores of 9. The researcher computes the mean and finds that the average score for the class is 9.85. The instructor concludes that the class can read what is written on the board. Then, as an afterthought, the instructor computes an internal-consistency measure of reliability. Shockingly, the reliability is .04. Is the test a reliable measure? Yes and no. No, it is a poor measure of individual differences. Yes, it can determine whether the class can read what is on the board. People can be highly accurate, but the test can be totally unreliable.

This confusion of the reliability of individual differences and the reliability of accuracy scores is nowhere more evident than in Crow and Hammond's (1957) Study 1. These investigators developed 15 different measures of accuracy. As they emphasized, these measures did not intercorrelate, which casts doubt on the reliability of the measures. Of the 12 measures for which it was possible to determine whether the subjects performed at better than chance levels, however, the subjects scored significantly above chance on 11. (The remaining measure showed significant performance *below* chance!) These data show remarkable levels of accuracy in the face of low reliability.

A second source of evidence of the limited individual differences in accuracy is in the area of nonverbal sensitivity. Individual differences in this area have proved to be elusive. The reliable measures — the Communication of Affect Receiving Ability Test (Buck, 1984) and the Profile of Nonverbal Sensitivity (Rosenthal, Hall, DiMatteo, Rogers, & Archer, 1979) — appear not to correlate with each other. Our (Kenny & La Voie, 1984) analysis indicated that individual differences in receiving and decoding ability are small. This analysis is independently supported by Bond, Kahler, and Paolicelli's (1985) data, which show individual differences in lie and truth detection to be modest. Also, attempts to improve people's skills in this area have not been very successful (Zuckerman, Koestner, & Alton, 1984) — a fact consistent with the view of minimal individual differences.

The final evidence concerns the studies that preceded the Cronbach critique. Certainly, a major reason why this researcher became interested in the accuracy issue was that studies showing individual differences in accuracy failed to replicate. This failure may not have been attributable so much to methodological shortcomings as to insufficient variance.

Therefore, in this chapter, individual differences are not given much attention; instead, the focus is nomothetic. The question is not who is accurate, but when and how people are accurate. Certainly there are individual differences in interpersonal accuracy. However, the variability of such differences is rather limited, and the study of the *level* of accuracy is likely to be more productive than the study of *variability*.

Interpersonal Orientation

Person perceivers in everyday life do not view their targets through one-way mirrors. They touch, yell at, and interact with each other. In a related vein, it is totally arbitrary to label one participant as the perceiver and the other as the target, because both people are usually judging each other (Tagiuri, 1969). Social perception is a two-sided experience. In a review of accuracy studies, Smith (1966, p. 26) noted that 56% of the studies involved judgments of targets with whom the perceivers had interacted. So social interaction is the rule, not the exception.

Swann (1984) has noted that interaction can enhance interpersonal accuracy. He has criticized the dominant use of object perception models in the field of person perception. One problem with object perception models is the assumption that the stimulus does not change when it is perceived by different perceivers. In person perception, a person's behavior can change when he or she interacts with different perceivers (see Chapter 1).

The argument that accuracy research should be interpersonal is not equivalent to Funder's (1987) argument that accuracy should be studied only in the real world. The issue is not *where* accuracy is studied; rather, it is *what type of stimulus* should be used to assess accuracy (real people with whom one can interact, as opposed to constructed verbal descriptions of people). The type of stimulus used in typical laboratory research in person perception can be found in the real world; one often makes judgments of individuals with whom one has not interacted. Thus, the mistakes or errors that people make in the laboratory would probably be made in the real world if the context in the real world were similar to that in the laboratory. But, to assess the accuracy of interpersonal perception, one should use an interactive context. This does not, however, preclude accuracy research in the laboratory, because interaction can occur in a laboratory context.

An interactive context is also important for methodological reasons. As reviewed in both Chapters 1 and 6, the basic questions in interpersonal perception are intertwined. First, there is reciprocity: If Al likes Bob, does Bob like Al? Second, there is assumed reciprocity: If Al likes Bob, does Al think that Bob likes Al? And third, there is accuracy: If Bob likes Al, does Art think that Bob likes Al? These three aspects can be viewed as forming a triangle. So if Al likes Bob and Bob likes Al (reciprocity), and Art also assumes that Bob likes Al (assumed reciprocity), then Art must be accurate at knowing that Bob likes Art. Thus, accuracy can be a by-product of reciprocity and assumed reciprocity. This potential confound can be measured and controlled only by studying both people in the dyad (see the discussion in Chapter 6 of dyadic meta-accuracy of affect). The second wave of accuracy research must allow for and take into account the two-sided nature of social perception.

Componential Orientation

The essence of the Cronbach and Gage critique is that judgments must not be treated globally, but must be broken down into components. Accuracy is measured by the correspondence between these components. Some of these components may largely tap the subjects' response set, and so correspondence between these components does not measure "true" accuracy.

Although they often pay lip service to the Cronbach and Gage critique in their introductions, many contemporary researchers compute global measures of accuracy in their results sections. Because the Cronbach and Gage critique occurred a generation ago, many contemporary accuracy researchers are unaware of the difficulties. Although there are notable exceptions (Harackiewicz & DePaulo, 1982), contemporary accuracy research is often not much better in methodology than pre-1955 research. Ironically, some pre-Cronbach articles—for example, the paper by Ausubel, Schiff, and Gasser (1952)—contain more sophisticated analyses than does a good deal of contemporary work. Modern accuracy researchers must seriously confront the Cronbach–Gage critique. Because researchers today have easy access to high-speed computers, the computational obstacles confronted by early researchers are no longer present.

Applying the Social Relations Model to Accuracy Research

If the second wave of accuracy research is to be nomothetic, interpersonal, and componential, it needs a new methodology. SRM can be applied to the study of accuracy and can be that new methodology (see Chapter 2).

In the Cronbach (1955) partitioning, the target × trait matrix (as in Table 7.1) is partitioned for each perceiver. Because the focus should be nomothetic, the partitioning that occurs within SRM is of the perceiver × target matrix for each trait. That is, the classical approach is to measure the accuracy for each perceiver across the set of targets and traits; the approach in this chapter is to measure the accuracy for a given trait across the set of perceivers and targets. Cronbach (1958) urged researchers not to measure accuracy across traits.

Because the focus is on the interpersonal nature of accuracy, the possibility that a person serves as both perceiver and target must be allowed. Also, the criterion score may be different for each perceiver. In prototypical accuracy research, the criterion does not change; that is, all perceivers' responses are compared with the same criterion score. But accuracy research needs to allow for the fact that the criterion score for the target may change for different perceivers (Swann, 1984).

Imagine two acquainted persons, Al and Bob. Each is asked to judge how competitive the other is. Al and Bob then interact in a structured situation (e.g., the Prisoner's Dilemma game), and both Al's and Bob's competitiveness is measured. These measurements are the criterion scores. Consider the question of how accurate Al is at judging how competitive Bob is.

As discussed in Chapter 2, in SRM, Al's judgment of Bob's competitiveness when interacting with Al is assumed to equal the following:

$$\begin{matrix} \text{Al's} & & & \text{Al's} & \text{Bob's} & \text{Al's} \\ \text{judgment} & = & \text{Constant} + & \text{perceiver} + & \text{target} + & \text{relationship} \\ \text{of Bob} & & & \text{effect} & \text{effect} & \text{effect with} \\ & & & & & \text{Bob} \end{matrix}$$

The terms of the equation are elaborated in Table 7.4.

The constant represents the average judgment of competitiveness across the set of perceivers and targets. The perceiver effect represents the average tendency for Al to believe that others are competitive. The target effect represents the tendency for perceivers to believe that Bob is competitive. The relationship effect measures the tendency for Al to believe that Bob is particularly competitive or cooperative when interacting with Al.

The criterion or behavioral score (how competitive Bob is when interacting with Al) can be partitioned into constant, actor, partner, and relationship. (The terms "perceiver" and "target" are not appropriate when behavior is being measured.) Its equation is as follows:

$$\begin{matrix} \text{Bob's} & & & \text{Bob's} & \text{Al's} & \text{Bob's} \\ \text{behavior} & = & \text{Constant} + & \text{actor} + & \text{partner} + & \text{relationship} \\ \text{with Al} & & & \text{effect} & \text{effect} & \text{effect with} \\ & & & & & \text{Al} \end{matrix}$$

These components are also elaborated in Table 7.4. The constant represents the tendency for targets to behave either competitively or cooperatively with their interaction partners. This term does not vary across perceivers or targets. The actor effect represents the tendency for Bob to behave competitively or cooperatively across all his interaction partners. The partner effect represents the extent to which Al's interaction partners generally behave competitively or cooperatively. And the relationship effect is the unique level of competitiveness in

TABLE 7.4. Components of the SRM Analysis of Target Accuracy

Al's rating of Bob's competitiveness (judgment)
    Constant: People's general rating of others' competitiveness
    Perceiver: Al's general prediction of others' competitiveness
    Target: Others' general rating of Bob's competitiveness
    Relationship: Al's rating of Bob's competitiveness, controlling for Al's perceiver
    effect and Bob's target effect

Bob's competitiveness with Al (criterion measure)
    Constant: People's general level of competitiveness
    Actor: Bob's general level of competitiveness
    Partner: Others' general level of competitiveness when interacting with Al
    Relationship: Bob's level of competitiveness when interacting with Al, con-
    trolling for Bob's actor effect and Al's partner effect

Note. Adapted from Kenny and Albright (1987). Copyright 1987 by the American Psychological Association. Adapted by permission.

Bob when he interacts with Al. The relationship effect is directional: Bob's unique level of competitiveness with Al may not match Al's unique level with Bob.

As in Figure 7.1 for the Cronbach components, accuracy in the SRM analysis can be conceptualized as the linking together of components; this is illustrated in Figure 7.2. As in the Cronbach analysis, there are four types of accuracy.

"Elevation accuracy" concerns the match between the perceivers' average response and the average response on the criterion measure. It is measured by the difference in the overall means (across perceivers and targets) between the judgment and the criterion. It is reasonable to measure elevation accuracy only if the two variables are expressed in the same unit of measurement.

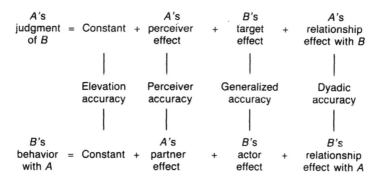

FIGURE 7.2. Four types of nomothetic accuracy. Adapted from Kenny and Albright (1987). Copyright 1987 by the American Psychological Association. Adapted by permission.

"Perceiver accuracy" (called "response set accuracy" in Kenny & Albright, 1987) concerns whether the perceiver's average response (perceiver effect on the judgment) corresponds to the average score of his or her interaction partners on the criterion (his or her partner effect on the criterion). Like stereotype accuracy in the Cronbach analysis (see note 4), perceiver accuracy may sometimes be informative. For instance, in the competitiveness example, people who expect their partners to be competitive may create that competitiveness via a self-fulfilling prophecy (see Chapter 10).

"Generalized accuracy" (called "individual accuracy" in Kenny & Albright, 1987) concerns the extent to which a person's behavior across interaction partners corresponds to how the individual is generally viewed. It measures the correlation between the target effect in the judgment and the actor effect in the criterion. In other words, it measures the correlation between how one is generally predicted to behave (the target effect in judgment) and how one actually behaves across interaction partners (the actor effect in the criterion). It is this type of accuracy that probably corresponds most closely to the naive notion of accuracy.

"Dyadic accuracy" concerns the ability of a perceiver to predict his or her partner's behavior, over and above the ability of other perceivers to predict the partner's behavior. It measures the correspondence between relationship components. For instance, in the competitiveness example, it measures a perceiver's ability to predict uniquely a given partner's competitive behavior with the perceiver. Can people differentially judge how individuals differentially behave with them?

The terms "generalized accuracy" and "dyadic accuracy" refer to the level of analysis and not to the specific content of the judgments. Generalized accuracy measures correspondence between others' judgments of a person and the behavior of that person. Thus, the analysis is at the individual level. Dyadic accuracy, on the other hand, measures the correspondence between differential judgments made by the perceiver and the differential behavior of a specific partner, and so it is at the dyadic level of analysis.

SRM's measures of accuracy are related to, but are not identical to, other formulations of accuracy. In a sense, generalized accuracy corresponds to differential elevation in the Cronbach system, and dyadic accuracy corresponds to Cronbach's differential accuracy. But this is only roughly the case, because in dyadic accuracy the issue is the accuracy for a trait across a set of perceivers and targets, whereas Cronbach examined the accuracy of a perceiver across a set of targets and traits (Kenny, 1981).

Swann (1984), as well as McHenry (1971), has defined two types of accuracy. Swann has defined "global accuracy" as the ability to predict how a person behaves in general with others, and "circumscribed accuracy" as the ability to predict the behavior of a person when in the presence of the perceiver. Swann's global accuracy corresponds to generalized accuracy, and his circumscribed accuracy corresponds to a combination of generalized and dyadic accuracy. If people know how someone behaves in general, they must know, at least in part, how the person behaves when interacting with them.

Before examining the accuracy correlations, one must first consider the variance partitioning. If there is no variance in the components of interest, it makes no sense to look at the correlations. For example, for people to achieve generalized accuracy, there must be actor variance in the criterion. That is, behavior must be consistent across interaction partners.

SRM's four types of accuracy are nomothetic: They measure accuracy for a given trait, as opposed to accuracy for a given perceiver. The model is also componential: The judgment and criterion are divided into components, and accuracy is measured by the correspondence between sets of components. Finally, it is interpersonal: A person can be both perceiver and target. SRM explicitly recognizes the two-sided nature of social interaction and can measure mutuality of social perceptions.

Criterion Measurement

The measurement of the components of accuracy is indeed complicated. There is, however, an even more difficult problem in accuracy research beyond the measurement of accuracy: the operationalization of the criterion. If Al thinks that Bob is competitive, how can it be ascertained whether Bob is truly competitive? Some researchers in person perception (e.g., Jones, 1985) have argued that problems of criterion measurement make accuracy research all but impossible.

How can a person's actual standing on a trait be known? Our earlier analysis (Kenny & Albright, 1987) identified five generic types of criterion measures: self-reports, expert judgments, mean judge ratings, operational criteria, and behavioral measurements. Each is considered here in turn.

Self-Reports

Self-reports are commonly used as the criterion measure in accuracy research. Sometimes a person is directly asked his or her standing on a trait, and in other instances self-report personality inventories are used to ascertain the person's standing. There are several problems with using self-report as a criterion measure. First, self-perception may be grossly distorted. People may be strongly motivated to present to themselves and to others favorable images of themselves. (See Chapter 9 for a more extended discussion of these biases.) Second, Wilson, Hull, and Johnson (1981) have shown that the self has less privileged access to information than might be thought. So why should the self be used as the standard? Third, when the perceiver and the self are acquainted, the self may try to persuade the other about his or her standing on the trait (Swann, 1990). So a perceiver who agrees with the self may be adopting the same mistaken view of the self. Researchers should, therefore, avoid using self-ratings as a criterion in *accuracy* research.

Nonetheless, the correlation between self- and other-ratings is an important question in interpersonal perception (though different from accuracy), and is a major topic in Chapter 9. There it is argued that other-perceptions are often a more valid measure than self-perceptions. (If this is true, it is more appropriate to validate self-ratings by other-ratings than vice versa!) It should be noted that if the perceiver is asked to rate a person as the person would rate himself or herself (i.e., to guess the person's self-perception), then the self-rating should be used as a criterion measure.

Expert Judgments

Expert judgments are made by someone who supposedly truly knows the target. For instance, a close friend of the target or the target's spouse may be used as an expert. In developmental research, the child's parent or teacher may be used as an expert. Because there is limited evidence that such people are any more accurate than nonexperts, researchers probably should avoid the use of so-called "expert" judgments as a criterion measure in accuracy research. Besides, expert judgments provide a measure of consensus and not a measure of accuracy. Moreover, as argued in Chapter 5, it is plausible that close friends and spouses may adopt relatively unique perspectives of the target.

Certainly, there are times when certain people do have specific knowledge about a target. For instance, teachers' ratings of aggressiveness may be used as a criterion measure for peers' ratings in a laboratory setting. In this instance, a teacher's rating is more akin to a behavioral rating than to an expert rating.

Mean Judgments

Sometimes researchers correlate a perceiver's ratings of targets with the average rating of the other perceivers. The use of mean judgment is problematic as a criterion in accuracy research, for much the same reason that expert judgments are problematic: If a perceiver's ratings correlate with the mean judgment, there is evidence of consensus and not accuracy. Mean judgments can be used to see who is *more* accurate (see the discussion of differential sensitivity in Chapter 5), but they cannot be used to establish the overall accuracy of judgment.

Operational Criteria

With an operational criterion, it is the *procedure* that guarantees the validity of the criterion measure. For instance, in clinical psychology "clinical insight" has been measured by having perceivers read suicide notes and then having the perceivers predict which people actually killed themselves. In social psychology, an operational criterion is often used in lie detection and deception research. Targets are instructed to tell two stories about an event, one true and the other false. The descriptions are videotaped and shown to perceivers. The task of the perceiver is to determine who told the truth and who lied. Operational criteria, although useful in studies of clinical insight and lie detection, are much less useful in determining the validity of traits. It is difficult to think of operational criteria for trait ratings.

Something akin to an operational criterion is an "event test" (Baron & Misovich, 1993). People are put into a situation that affords the utilization of the trait. For instance, it is easier to study extroversion at a party than in a library. However, an event test is more appropriately viewed as a behavioral criterion than as an operational criterion.

Behavioral Observations

In a behavioral observation, observers watch the target engage in behavior and then rate the target's behavior. Behavioral judgment is very costly and time-consuming, and behavioral measures often show poor test–retest consistency, but behavioral ratings are often the best possible way to measure the person's actual standing on a trait.

When observers are asked to rate behavior, the scales should be made as objective as possible. For instance, instead of rating friendliness, observers should count or measure the duration of smiles. When behavior ratings are thus made specific, there may be the consequent problem of linking the behavior to the trait being rated. For example, how is it known that smiling indicates friendliness, given that there is evidence that smiling sometimes indicates deception?

In addition to not using global ratings, researchers should attempt to establish high levels of interrater reliability. That is, to show that the behavior ratings are relatively objective, different raters should agree with one another.

Behavioral measurement typically requires recording the target by videotape or audiotape, as well as obtaining informed consent, so that the interactants know that they are being recorded. Such knowledge may distort a person's behavior. Targets may behave unnaturally when they know that they are being recorded, because they are objectively self-aware. Fortunately, in this day and age of hand-held video recorders, this self-awareness caused by video recording is probably less problematic.

Choice of a Criterion Measure

Researchers need to use good judgment in deciding what problems there are with a given criterion measure. There are many contexts where self-ratings are serviceable. For instance, most of the early studies of zero acquaintance used self-ratings. There are certainly going to be cases in which behavioral observations are not practical (Zebrowitz, 1990). Moreover, there are going to be instances in which expert ratings and self-ratings are valid. Although my own preference is for behavioral observations, it is necessary to have an open mind in designing research.

These difficulties in developing a criterion measure are the most significant obstacle in accuracy research (Jones, 1985). They have led some to conclude that accuracy research is just impossible, and have led others (Kruglanski, 1989) to conclude that all accuracy research is only consensus research—in other words, that accuracy research always involves comparing one set of person perceptions to another set. Every type of criterion measure (except perhaps an operational criterion) can be viewed as a person perception. Even a behavioral rating is still a person perception, because observers still code the behaviors. Although this view has considerable validity, there is good reason to believe that some ratings are closer to the target's actual standing than are others. Moreover, this same criticism applies equally well to "objective" physical measures: They all require human judgment. Ever since Einstein, scientists have realized that there is always an element of subjectivity in measurement.

Once a criterion measure has been developed, it may still be necessary to make an important modification in that measure. Because a person's behavior may change when the person interacts with different partners, the criterion score may well vary for each person making a prediction. As Swann (1984) has emphasized, accuracy researchers need to know how the person behaves with each person who makes predictions. So, if possible, the researcher should try to measure the criterion dyadically.

Examples of Accuracy Research

In this section, I consider two specific applications of SRM to the accuracy question. The first considers people's ability to remember how frequently they interact with others. Accuracy in this case would not be very surprising. The second study concerns people's ability to predict the behavior of their interaction partners based on minimal information. Accuracy in this case would be very impressive.

Do You Know Whom You Were with Last Friday?

In an important series of studies, Bernard, Killworth, and Sailer (1982) asked people in four different contexts with whom they spent time. The four groups were members of a college fraternity (Frat), workers in an office at a company (Office), a technical work group (Tech), and a group of ham radio operators (Ham). Bernard et al. kept track over a period of time of how frequently the people in each group interacted with one another. The investigators then asked people to recall how frequently they interacted during the period of observation. So the judgment was the estimated frequency of interaction, and the criterion was the actual amount of interaction based on behavioral observation. In two of the four studies (Office and Tech), the judgment task was to rank-order the others in terms of frequency of interaction.

A colleague and I (Kashy & Kenny, 1990a) reanalyzed these four data sets. In these studies, it was possible to measure three of the four types of accuracy depicted in Figure 7.2. (It was not possible to measure elevation accuracy, because the judgment and criterion had different units of measurement.) Perceiver accuracy concerns the following question: Does a person know how frequently he or she interacts with others? Perceiver accuracy could not be measured in two of the studies because ranking was used in the judgments. Generalized accuracy concerns the following question: Does a person know how much he or she interacts with others? Finally, dyadic accuracy concerns the following question: Does a person know how frequently he or she especially interacts with a given person?

The results from the analyses of these four studies are contained in Table 7.5. They show little evidence for perceiver accuracy, and strong evidence for generalized accuracy and dyadic accuracy. It should be noted that the dyadic-accuracy correlations are not disattenuated (see Chapter 2), and so it should not be concluded that there is more generalized than dyadic accuracy. The interested reader should consult Kashy and Kenny (1990a) for more details.

Behavioral Predictions of Extroversion at Zero Acquaintance

Can people predict how others will behave on the basis of minimal information? Most of us probably would think not; however, as reviewed in Chapter 4, there is a remarkable amount of consensus of judgment at zero acquaintance, particularly on the factor of Extroversion. Moreover, as reviewed in Chapter 9, these judgments at zero acquaintance predict self-ratings. Thus, if a judge believes that someone is extroverted, that person probably sees himself or herself as extroverted. So there is the rather strong possibility that consensual judgments made at zero acquaintance are valid. A colleague and I (Levesque & Kenny, 1993) set out to see whether this was so.

We brought 20 groups of four women into the laboratory. We first made sure that they were unacquainted with one another. We then asked each woman, in front of the other three women, to state her

TABLE 7.5. Correlational Measures of Three Types of Accuracy, Based on Data from Bernard et al. (1982)

Study	Perceiver	Generalized	Dyadic
Frat	.08	.81	.43
Office	—[a]	.58	.42
Tech	—[a]	.75	.48
Ham	.72	.97	.46

Note. Adapted from Kashy and Kenny (1990a). Copyright 1990 by the American Sociological Association. Adapted by permission.
[a]Correlation cannot be computed because rankings were used.

name, her year in college, her hometown, and where she currently lived at school. Next, we had the four women rate one another on the Big Five factors. We obtained the usual result of consensus on Extroversion (target variance of 26%) and little or no consensus on the other four factors (an average of 3%).

The next stage of the study involved behavioral predictions. We asked each woman to predict the behavior of the other three women in each of the following categories: talkativeness, gestures, nervousness, voice animation, and body lean. We asked each woman to make predictions of how the other women would behave with her and how they would behave with others. It turned out that there was virtually no difference between the two types of predictions. The women thought that the other women would behave basically the same way with them as with other people. We also found that all of the predictions were strongly correlated with Extroversion judgments. In essence, if perceivers thought that the targets were extroverted, they thought that the targets would engage in more behaviors. They did, however, think that the targets who were extroverted would be *less* nervous.

In the next phase, we had the women interact dyadically for 5 minutes per interaction. We videotaped both interactants in each instance, and these videotapes were coded by trained judges whose judgments were averaged. Generally high levels of agreement were obtained. The reliabilities ranged from .66 for nervousness to .99 for percentage of time gesturing. Levesque and I partitioned the variance of the behavioral ratings and found strong evidence for both actor and relationship effects in these ratings. Consistent with previous work (Kenny & Malloy, 1988), there was little or no evidence of partner effects in the behavioral data.

The components of the behavioral ratings were then correlated with the initial predictions of talking, gesturing, nervousness, voice tone, and body lean. The correlations, presented in Table 7.6, provide very strong evidence that the predictions were indeed accurate; however, accuracy was limited to generalized accuracy. That is, women who were predicted by everyone to be nervous or talkative were perceived as nervous or talkative by their interaction partners.

The Levesque and Kenny (1993) study provides very strong evidence that Extroversion judgments made at zero acquaintance are valid. It also indicates that global or generalized accuracy is much greater than circumscribed or dyadic accuracy. Swann's (1984) hypothesis to the contrary needs testing in cases where people know one another better.

TABLE 7.6. Accuracy Correlations of Behavior with Predictions

Behavior	Perceiver	Generalized	Dyadic
Talkativeness	##	.56	.03
Nervousness	##	.55	−.06
Body lean	##	.47	.04
Voice animation	##	.92	−.05
Gestures	##	.50	−.03

Note. ## = insufficient variance (less than 10%) to compute correlation. Adapted from Levesque and Kenny (1993). Copyright 1993 by the American Psychological Association. Adapted by permission.

Accuracy and the Weighted-Average Model

In Chapter 4, a general mathematical model of perception called WAM has been proposed. In that chapter, as well as Chapter 5, WAM has been used only to study agreement and disagreement. In this section, the primary question is as follows: What is the relationship between accuracy and acquaintance?

In WAM, perception is assumed to be based on the behavior of the target, the physical appearance of the target (stereotypes), and the unique impression that the perceiver has of the target. Moreover, two different perceivers may influence each other's perception of the target. The reader may find it helpful to review the model parameters presented in Chapter 4 before reading the following sections.

Choice of Criterion

As reviewed earlier in this chapter, one very difficult problem in the study of accuracy is the selection of a criterion measure. The assumption I have made (Kenny, 1991) is that the criterion is a theoretical average of all possible behaviors viewed by all possible perceivers. Following Kruglanski (1989), this definition of the criterion recognizes that accuracy is ultimately a form of consensus.

Because this theoretical criterion is an average across all possible behaviors, the effects of physical appearance or unique impression are overwhelmed by behavioral information. The criterion score for a target is a *theoretical* impression of all possible perceivers examining all possible behaviors. In practice, it is never observed, but with WAM, the correlation between perception and this theoretical value can be computed.

Accuracy and Acquaintance

WAM (see Appendix C) can be used to describe the relationship between acquaintance and target accuracy. Overlap, which so dramatically affects consensus, has virtually no effect on the target accuracy of a single rater. Overlap affects accuracy only when there is communication: Communication results in greater accuracy when there is *less* overlap, because with less overlap the two perceivers gain more information about the target from the communication.

Generally, increasing acquaintance leads to increasing target accuracy. So, unlike consensus, increasing acquaintance leads to greater accuracy. There are two important exceptions to this rule. First, there must be some degree of consistency in the target's behavior (i.e., r_1 must be greater than zero). If there were no consistency at all, there would be no accuracy. Second, the "kernel of truth" parameter, or r_4, cannot be too high. If there is a sufficient level of "kernel of truth" in the stereotypes, then the relationship between accuracy and acquaintance is concave (U-shaped): Increasing acquaintance leads to an initial decline in accuracy, and then as acquaintance increases, accuracy increases. But even when there is a "kernel of truth," at some point with increasing acquaintance there is greater accuracy.

If there is no communication, as acquaintance increases, the limit of accuracy is the square root of the parameter of similar meaning systems. So the different meaning systems that perceivers have place a severe limit on a person's accuracy as it also does on consensus. Park, DeKay, and Kraus (1994) estimate the meaning-systems correlation as about .4. So the limit on the accuracy correlation for an individual's perception may be about .65.

Classical psychometric theory states that validity is the square root of reliability. To translate this statement into WAM's terms, accuracy is the square root of consensus. This holds within WAM when each of the three following conditions holds: there is no overlap ($q = 0$), there is no agreement about stereotypes ($r_3 = 0$), and there is no communication ($a = 0$). Because these conditions do not generally hold, and when they are violated consensus is greater than the square root of the validity, consensus is likely to be a very misleading index of accuracy.

Given that target behaviors are consistent, accuracy should increase with increasing acquaintance. However, as reviewed in Chapter 4, there is not a very close relationship between consensus and acquaintance. So consensus cannot be used as a proxy measure of accuracy. Therefore, a longitudinal study should reveal little or no increase in consensus but an increase in target accuracy.

WAM, at least as currently formulated, fails to consider Swann's (1984) hypothesis that a perceiver may be accurate at predicting the behavior of a target when that target interacts with the perceiver, but the perceiver may not be accurate in predicting the target's interactions with others. Perhaps some modification of WAM's definition of the criterion is necessary to allow for what Swann (1984) calls "circumscribed accuracy."

Conclusion

It seems hard to believe that such a simple question — Do people know what others are like? — is such a difficult question to answer. This seemingly simple question has proved to be so complex that some social and personality psychologists have given up trying to answer it.

The question is difficult in two distinct ways. First, a single accuracy question cannot be asked (e.g., Are people accurate?); rather, the judgment and criterion must be partitioned into components, and multiple accuracy questions must be asked. Second, it is difficult, but not impossible, to ascertain what a person is really like. Even the best possible type of criterion measure, behavioral ratings, is still a collection of person perceptions. Despite all of these difficulties, accuracy research is still worth all of the trouble because it is a central question in interpersonal perception. For instance, there is currently considerable debate as to whether depressives are more or less accurate person perceivers than are nondepressives.

This chapter presents the results from two studies that do show that people are accurate. They do know with whom they spend time, especially at the dyadic level, and they can predict how their interaction partners will behave. Thus, the evidence for target accuracy from these initial studies is quite impressive. Social science is beginning to see that the view of the person perceiver as a biased and faulty perceiver is not complete. The person perceiver is perhaps more like the bumbling Peter Sellers as Inspector Clouseau than the omniscient Raymond Burr as Perry Mason, but in the end they both "get their man."

Considerable empirical and theoretical research about accuracy must still be conducted. Perhaps the most difficult challenge that presents itself is the development of the linkages between observable behaviors and traits (Trope & Higgins, 1993). That is, what behaviors correspond to what trait judgments? Also, Swann's (1984) hypothesis that perceivers are better able to predict their partners' behavior with them than with others has never been empirically demonstrated. Nor do we have any evidence that people are especially accurate at predicting the behavior of someone with whom they are close. These and other questions await the curiosity of interested researchers. We have the methodology to tackle accuracy research; there is no longer any excuse for ignoring the phenomenon.

The next chapter also considers the accuracy question, but it concerns the accuracy of meta-perception, not of other-perception.

Notes

1. Of course, sometimes perceivers may be better off if they do not know the truth (Steiner, 1955). For example, bosses may not need to know how their employees really feel about them, and parents may not need to know the truth about their adolescents' sexual behavior.

2. In 1958, Cronbach developed an approach entirely different from the one in his 1955 article. He emphasized analyzing trait by trait instead of computing accuracy across the set of traits. So the expression "Cronbach analysis" as I use it here refers to his 1955 article, and not to his views since 1958.

3. For all but elevation, Cronbach (1955) discussed two aspects of accuracy. The first, the correlation between the judgment component and the criterion component, has been discussed here. The second concerns the reduction in variance of the judgments, given the degree of correlation between the judgment and the criterion. This variance reduction is especially important when the judges are using the same unit of measurement as the criterion. Because this is often not the case, the correlational measure of accuracy and not the variance reduction measure is discussed.

4. There are circumstances in which stereotype accuracy should be considered as "true" accuracy. It may reflect sensitivity to the generalized other (Bronfenbrenner, Harding, & Gallwey, 1958).

5. The study by Cline and Richards (1960) is frequently cited as a post-Cronbach study showing the generalizability of indiviudal differences. In a subsequent article, however, Richards and Cline (1963) noted that they had made a mistake in their measure of differential accuracy. The proper measures of differential accuracy show modest correlations with other measures of accuracy.

Chapter 8

META-PERCEPTION

W hat do others think of us? How do we know? When people form a judgment about what others think of them, are people likely to be right? A colleague and I reviewed issues of meta-perception and meta-accuracy (Kenny & DePaulo, 1993), and this chapter summarizes the results of our review.

Theoretical Review

The importance and interest value of issues in person perception, unlike those of many questions posed by social scientists, are immediately apparent even to the layperson. Other people clearly are not passive objects; when we perceive them, they perceive us in return. Not surprisingly, then, people try to perceive others' perceptions of them. They try to "get into other people's heads" and "read their minds." That people are motivated to predict and control their worlds is an assumption that few psychologists would deny. Certainly, accurate perceptions are useful in knowing whether the hand behind another person's back holds a gift or a weapon. The question of whether people know how others view them has held a position of prominence in clinical psychology, personality psychology, and social psychology, and it has also been accorded special importance in sociology.

Views from Different Disciplines

Sociology

In sociology, the symbolic-interactionist position, set forth in the ground-breaking work of Mead (1925, 1934) and Cooley (1902), pro-

This chapter is adapted from Kenny and DePaulo (1993). Copyright 1993 by the American Psychological Association. Adapted by permission.

poses that our very selves are a product of our perceptions of how others view us (Shrauger & Schoeneman, 1979). Cooley (1902) coined the term "looking-glass self" to describe the process by which a person looks into the eyes and minds of others and imagines how those others view him or her. Symbolic interactionists assume that meta-perceptions (which are called "reflected appraisals") are usually accurate (Kinch, 1963). It is one purpose of this chapter to evaluate that assumption empirically.

According to the symbolic-interactionist tradition, people can look into two kinds of minds in their quest to learn how others view them. There are the minds of specific other people, usually significant others (Cooley, 1902); there is also the mind of the "generalized other" (Mead, 1934). When people look into the mind of the generalized other, they are trying to determine "the generalized standpoint of the social group as a whole" (Mead, 1934, p. 138). In this chapter, there is a comparison between people's ability to read the minds of specific others and their ability to read the mind of the generalized other.

Clinical Psychology

In clinical psychology, the question of whether people know how others view them has been deemed important, in part because of the assumption that often people do not know (e.g., Smith, 1966). Depressed people, for example, can be relentless in their insistence that no one likes them. For a long time, it was believed that depressed people are harder on themselves than they should be (e.g., Beck, 1967). More recently, however, that view has been challenged by the provocative suggestion that depressed people are right after all. According to this "sadder but wiser" perspective, depressives' gloomy assessments of how others view them are right on target; nondepressed people, with their overly optimistic views of how others see them, are the ones who are inaccurate (e.g., Lewinsohn, Mischel, Chaplin, & Barton, 1980). The controversy continues to rage (e.g., Alloy & Abramson, 1988; Campbell & Fehr, 1990). At the heart of this debate are issues addressed in this chapter: How should researchers measure accuracy, and how do laypeople attain it?

Personality Psychology

Among the people who care most deeply about what others think of them are those who are socially anxious or shy, and those who are dependent on the approval of others. Personality psychologists have been intensely interested in these kinds of individuals and have learned much about them. For example, they have shown that socially anxious people—those who want very much to convey particular impressions of themselves to others, but are insecure about their ability to do so (e.g., Leary, 1983; Schlenker & Leary, 1982)—think that others take an especially dim view of them, even in experimental research in which the feedback they receive is identical to that received by individuals who are not socially anxious (Pozo, Carver, Wellens, & Scheier, 1991).

People high in need for approval are evaluatively dependent, and they are highly motivated to be viewed favorably by others (Crowne & Marlowe, 1960). Unlike socially anxious people, individuals who are high in the need for approval describe themselves in glowing rather than derogatory terms. Such self-descriptions, however, may be more defensive than accurate. Both individual differences may be important predictors of the ways in which people think they are viewed by others.

Social Psychology

In social psychology, the question of whether people know how they are viewed by others has been central to at least two traditions: the self-presentational perspective on human behavior, and the study of accuracy of person perception. Self-presentational perspectives assume that people often try to convey particular impressions of themselves to others (e.g., Baumeister, 1982; DePaulo, 1992; Goffman, 1959; Jones, 1964; Schlenker, 1980, 1985; Snyder, 1979; Tedeschi, 1981). The success of these attempts may depend on the skillful monitoring of the reactions of others. If it appears that others are forming an impression other than the desired one, then self-presentation efforts and strategies can then be modified accordingly.

The accuracy tradition is one of the oldest in the fields of social and personality psychology (Jones, 1990; Kenny & Albright, 1987). As reviewed in Chapter 7, much of the work in this area has been concerned with other-perceptions, which are the judgments that people make about the traits and other attributes of other people. A key question is whether people can predict how others describe themselves: For example, does Jack know how Jill sees herself? But questions about meta-perceptions (Laing, Phillipson, & Lee, 1966)—judgments of how others view us—have been important, too.

When Are Meta-Perceptions Accurate?

Both the symbolic-interactionist and the self-presentational perspectives can be construed as arguing that people always care about how they are viewed by others. Even if meta-perception is taken to be a fact of social life, there are certain to be variations in the intensity of people's yearning to know what others are thinking of them. Outcome dependence may be the most important predictor of this yearning. When people believe that their outcomes are determined by another person's impression of them, they should be highly motivated to discern, monitor, and control that impression. Persons of low status or power, then, may be more invested in meta-perceiving their high-status interaction partners than vice versa (e.g., Snodgrass, 1985, 1992).

Motivation alone, however, does not guarantee that meta-perceptions are accurate (Kruglanski, 1989). If we are to learn something about others' view of us by looking into their eyes, there must be something worth seeing there—something that is not misleading or not so subtle that it is likely to be missed. Are there valid cues to others' impressions in everyday face-to-face social interactions? Are we likely to be able to read those cues?

Research on nonverbal communication in very controlled settings suggests that people are accurate at reading cues such as facial expressions, voice tones, and body movements, and that this accuracy exceeds chance levels for children as well as adults (e.g., DePaulo & Rosenthal, 1982). Many studies clearly indicate that people *can* understand nonverbal cues under particular circumstances. But spontaneous face-to-face interactions may create very different circumstances. The kinds of nonverbal behaviors that occur in everyday social life are typically much less clear than those that comprise standardized stimulus materials. Furthermore, many cues are available in social interactions other than nonverbal ones, and interactants have a variety of tasks to contend with other than monitoring one another's nonverbal behaviors. This cognitive "busyness" seems to foster a bit of naiveté, and so people who have many tasks (such as planning their own performances in addition to monitoring other people's) may be especially likely to take what they hear and see at face value (Gilbert, 1991).

Moreover, people are probably only rarely entirely straightforward about how they feel about one another. Besides instances of outright deception, there is also much omission. That people are reluctant to convey bad news has been amply demonstrated (Swann, Stein-Seroussi, & McNulty, 1992; Tesser & Rosen, 1975). What is even more interesting is that people can also be reluctant to convey good news when it is in the form of explicit evaluations of others' personalities (e.g., Blumberg, 1972; Felson, 1980).

The information that is available to people, then, about what others think of them may not be all that plentiful or clear. Even if people care deeply about discerning others' *true* impressions of them, the task can be quite challenging (DePaulo, Stone, & Lassiter, 1985). But people may more often wish to see in the mirror of others' eyes a reflection that makes them feel good about themselves, or one that confirms what they already feel is true of themselves (e.g., Swann, 1990).

The question of interest is whether people attend to, and process insightfully and even-handedly, information about how others view them that is available during ongoing social interactions. Because natural and spontaneous interactions are of interest, the strategy of experimentally manipulating the cues that are available to people to determine how they use such cues (e.g., DePaulo, Rosenthal, Eisenstat, Rogers, & Finkelstein, 1978) is not entirely serviceable in the initial stages of this research. Instead, the evidence comes from more indirect patterns of findings. For example, if people are attending carefully to cues from others about the kinds of impressions that they are conveying, then they are likely to think that they convey different impressions to different people—particularly if they interact with each of those different people separately and at different times. They may also notice that particular people form unique impressions of them. For instance, Jack may notice that Jill sees him differently than she sees anyone else, and that he is seen differently by Jill than he is seen by anyone else. Furthermore, if people are attending faithfully to other people's cues, then their meta-perceptions of how others view them should match how others say they really do view them. That is, their meta-perceptions should be accurate. And they should be accurate not just in the general sense (e.g., popular people know they are popular), but also in the more differentiated sense (they know which particular people find them particularly lovable).

This chapter focuses on interpersonal perception processes that occur on-line during social interactions. These are of special interest because they are the raw data of social life. But people interested in how others view them sometimes have other kinds of information available to them, too. For example, there are third-person communications: Jim can tell Jack how much Jill likes him (Felson, 1980). Or, if Jim does not volunteer this information, Jack can send Frank out as a "spy" to try to find out what Jill thinks of Jack (Felson, 1980). And of course, numerous cues are available from the partners themselves. Jill, for instance, may or may not stare into Jack's eyes, ask him whether he would like to take a walk up the hill with her, or tumble after him if he falls down the hill. Even these kinds of cues can be ambiguous, and so even when they are available, meta-accuracy can be quite difficult to achieve.

Meta-Perception as Self-Perception

Given the difficulty of monitoring a partner's reactions in social inter-action, people may use other sources of information to form meta-perceptions. People can, without looking at the behaviors or the reac-tions of others, examine their own behaviors and imagine how the other person may view these. This is akin to the self-perception process. Ac-cording to self-perception theory (Bem, 1967), perceivers sometimes observe their overt behavior to infer their own internal states, such as their opinions and preferences. In the version that is proposed here, people observe their own behavior to discern what others may be think-ing of them.

As Felson (1981, 1992) has noted, the process can be a bit more complicated than that. People may observe their own behavior and form their own judgments (self-perceptions) of that behavior. Then they may assume that others would judge their behavior as they do. Instead of inferring directly from their own behavior how others view them (as in the simple model), they form their own impressions first, then assume that other people's impressions would be similar.

In some circumstances, people's self-perceptions of their own be-havior may be nearly identical to their self-concept. This may happen if people tend to develop strongly held beliefs about what they are really like, and if they think that these identity-defining characteristics (their "true" personalities, as they see them) are immediately apparent to others. So, for example, a woman who sees herself as kind, generous, and able to make others feel at ease may think that these qualities are evident in all of her behaviors, even those occurring during brief in-teractions with total strangers. She does not think that she needs to observe her own behaviors or other people's reactions to her own be-haviors; she knows what she is like, and she is sure that when others meet her, they will know too.

To learn whether people know what kinds of impressions they make on others, and how they make these determinations, we must examine meta-perception processes as they occur across a variety of interaction partners. For if we look only at Jack and Jill and ask whether Jack can tell how Jill perceives him, and we find that Jack's meta-perception does in fact seem similar to Jill's actual impression of him, we cannot know on that basis alone why Jack's meta-perception is simi-lar to Jill's actual perception. Perhaps Jack always thinks that he makes that sort of impression; in other words, his meta-perception in this instance may have nothing to do with Jill in particular. Or perhaps Jill is the sort of person who makes everyone feel loved, in which case Jack's feeling of being loved may have nothing to do with him in particular. Or perhaps there really is something special about the particular way that Jill perceives Jack, and Jack does indeed know this.

An important feature of the research design, then, is that each subject interacts with and is judged by multiple partners. Each person in each study serves as both subject and partner; thus, the interactions are characterized by the mutuality and interdependence that typify social life. These kinds of studies are extremely labor-intensive, and the Social Relations Model (SRM) analysis that is so well suited to this type of investigation has only recently been developed (Kenny & La Voie, 1984). Eight studies fit all of the criteria and are reviewed in this chapter. Four of the eight are 1990s studies, and three more were conducted in the 1980s.

Applying the Social Relations Model to Meta-Perception Research

In this chapter, SRM, as presented in Chapter 2, is used to analyze perceptions and meta-perceptions. The use of the model provides a more detailed look at meta-perceptions and meta-accuracy. An example in which Jack and Jill interact is used throughout this chapter. Jill forms an impression of Jack, and Jack then attempts to infer Jill's impression of him. Jill is symbolized by L and Jack by K. According to SRM, Jill's impression of Jack (which is an other-perception of him, not a meta-perception) depends on these three components:

1. Perceiver: how Jill views people in general, or $L(↑)$.
2. Target: how Jack is generally viewed by others, or $↑(K)$.
3. Relationship: how Jill uniquely views Jack, or $l(k)$.

The meta-perception of how Jack thinks Jill views him can be correspondingly decomposed:

4. Perceiver: how Jack thinks others see him, or $K(↑(K))$.
5. Target: how others think that Jill views people, or $↑(L(↑))$.
6. Relationship: how Jack thinks that Jill uniquely views him, or $k(l(k))$.

As described in Chapters 2 and 7, within SRM there are two different types of meta-accuracy: generalized and dyadic meta-accuracy. "Generalized meta-accuracy" describes people's ability to understand how they are generally viewed by others. It is their sensitivity to the ways in which they are regarded by a group of people as a whole, apart from the ways in which they may be viewed differently by different members of the group. Generalized accuracy[1] is the correlation of the target effect in the impression or other-perception (e.g., how Jack is viewed by others) with the perceiver effect of the meta-perception (e.g., how Jack thinks he is viewed by others). Thus, generalized meta-accuracy is the correlation between components 2 and 4 in the list above, and is symbolized by $\Lambda(K) = K(\Lambda(K))$.

"Dyadic meta-accuracy" describes people's ability to know how they are differentially regarded by particular other people. Dyadic accuracy implies that people can tell which particular other people have especially favorable or unfavorable impressions of them. Dyadic accuracy is the correlation between the relationship effects of both variables, or the correlation between components 3 and 6 in the list above; it is symbolized by $l(k) = k(l(k))$.

In studies in which there are multiple replications (i.e., the judge is rated by the target on two or more variables or at two or more times), it is possible to separate an unstable or time-specific effect from a stable relationship effect. For those studies, the effect attributable to relationship with the unstable effect removed ("dyadic adjusted") is presented.

Research Evidence

Table 8.1 presents a brief description of the eight studies we reviewed (Kenny & DePaulo, 1993). For each study, the measures were separated into types: trait and affect (usually liking and disliking). If there were multiple measures, the correlations were averaged.

Variance Partitioning

Traits

When Jill sees Jack as good-natured and smart, to what extent may she do so because she tends to see everyone as good-natured and smart? These perceiver variances in perceptions of traits are presented in the first column of Table 8.2, and they are substantial. The results across studies indicate that people do seem to view others in consistent ways (e.g., they see all people as good-natured and smart). There is also substantial perceiver variance across studies in meta-perceptions. That is, people think they make a consistent impression on all of the targets (e.g., they think that the targets generally view them as good-natured and smart). The first conclusion, then, is that there is

TABLE 8.1. Study Descriptions

Anderson (1985)
  Number of groups: 5, same-sex
  Number of subjects: 121
  Setting or task; acquaintance: Residential; long-term
  Variables: Humorous, intelligent, considerate, defensive

Curry & Emerson (1970)
  Number of groups: 6, 4 all-male and 2 all-female
  Number of subjects: 48
  Setting or task; acquaintance: Residential; long-term (1–8 weeks)
  Variables: Affect

DePaulo, Kenny, Hoover, Webb, & Oliver (1987)
  Number of groups: 7
  Number of subjects: 42 females
  Setting or task; acquaintance: One-on-one interactions; none
  Variables: Competence and affect

Kenny & DePaulo (1990)
  Number of groups: 8
  Number of subjects: 48
  Setting or task; acquaintance: Three interviewers questioning an
    opposite-sex applicant for a residential assistant position; none
  Variables: Competence and affect

Malloy & Albright (1990)
  Number of groups: 21, same-sex
  Number of subjects: 84
  Setting or task; acquaintance: Residential; long-term
  Variables: Sociable, good-natured, responsible, calm, intelligent

Malloy & Janowski (1992)
  Number of groups: 10, mixed-sex
  Number of subjects: 68
  Setting or task; acquaintance: Group discussions to consensus; none
  Variables: Leadership and quality of ideas

Oliver (1989)
  Number of groups: 14
  Number of subjects: 56
  Setting or task; acquaintance: One-on-one, male–female "first date" inter-
    actions; none
  Variables: Activity and affect

Reno & Kenny (1992)
  Number of groups: 20, all-female
  Number of subjects: 102
  Setting or task; acquaintance: One-on-one interactions; none
  Variables: Information conveyed, open, private, trust, likable

Note. Adapted from Kenny and DePaulo (1993). Copyright 1993 by the American Psychological Association. Adapted by permission.

TABLE 8.2. Variance Partitioning of Trait Studies

Study	Perceiver	Target	Relationship	Error	Rel./err.
Anderson (1985)					
Trait	—	.33	—	—	.67
Meta-perception	.40	.03	—	—	.57
DePaulo et al. (1987)					
Trait	.37	.07	.18	.38	—
Meta-perception	.54	.03	.09	.34	—
Kenny & DePaulo (1990)					
Applicant					
Trait	.19	.35	.15	.30	—
Meta-perception	.69	.01	.03	.28	—
Interviewer					
Trait	.58	.06	.05	.31	—
Meta-perception	.75	.00	.01	.24	—
Malloy & Albright (1990)					
Trait	.21	.34	—	—	.45
Meta-perception	.68	.03	—	—	.29
Malloy & Janowski (1992)					
Trait	.06	.45	.24	.25	—
Meta-perception	.37	.01	.28	.35	—
Oliver (1989)					
Trait	.13	.62	—	—	.24
Meta-perception	.56	.21	—	—	.23
Reno & Kenny (1992)					
Trait	.30	.12	—	—	.57
Meta-perception	.44	.02	—	—	.55
Mean					
Trait	.26	.29	.16	.31	.48
Meta-perception	.55	.04	.10	.30	.41

Note. For Kenny and DePaulo (1990), the "Trait" entries under "Applicant" refer to the interviewers' impressions of the applicants' traits. The "Meta-perception" entries indicate the applicants' beliefs about how they were viewed by others. Similarly, the "Trait" entries under "Interviewer" indicate the applicants' impressions of the interviewers, and the "Meta-perception" entries indicate the interviewers' beliefs about how they were perceived by the applicants. Adapted from Kenny and DePaulo (1993). Copyright 1993 by the American Psychological Association. Adapted by permission.

perceiver variance in both perceptions and meta-perceptions of traits: People view others in consistent ways, and they think that they are viewed by others in consistent ways.

Second, when perceiver variances are compared, there is a very strong tendency for these variances to be much larger for meta-perceptions than for trait perceptions. In all seven of the possible comparisons, the perceiver variance is larger for meta-perception than for the direct or trait perception. On average across the studies, 29% more variance is attributable to perceiver for meta-perception than for trait perceptions, and the median level of perceiver variance for meta-perceptions is 55%. These results indicate that people tend to see others in certain consistent ways (e.g., as generally good-natured or smart). But there is even more consistency in the ways that they think they are viewed by other people; for example, they may think that they generally convey an impression of kindness or competence to the many different kinds of people with whom they interact. This belief exists across all levels of acquaintance. It is true in studies in which Jack and Jill and Jack's many other friends have lived together for weeks or even months, and it is also true for the studies in which Jack and each of his Jills have scaled the hill for the first time.

If Jack thinks that Jill sees him as good-natured and smart, is that perhaps in part because Jill seems to see everyone that way? Interestingly, there is very little target variance in meta-perceptions. The median proportion across studies is only .03, and the most parsimonious interpretation is that there is no target variance in meta-perceptions. Only the Oliver (1989) study shows evidence of target variance. The failure to find target variance in meta-perceptions indicates that there is no consistent tendency for certain people to be seen as harsh evaluators and others as lenient. In contrast, there is evidence of target variance in other-perceptions. This indicates that particular targets are viewed in consistent ways by different perceivers. As reviewed in Chapter 4, trait perceptions are consensual.

Is there something special about the way that Jill views Jack—something unique to her perceptions of Jack? And is there something special about the way Jack thinks he is viewed by Jill? The answers to these questions are to be found in the relationship variance. Relationship variance in other-perceptions occurs when people form unique impressions of particular others. Relationship variance in meta-perceptions occurs when people think that they are viewed differently by different people. In four of the studies (all involving short-term acquaintances), it is possible to separate relationship from error variance. These studies indicate some tendency, though it is not very strong, for people to form unique impressions of particular other people. That

is, there is some small amount of relationship variance in trait perceptions. The amount of relationship variance in meta-perceptions is even
smaller. In three of the four comparisons, there is less relationship variance for meta-perceptions than for other-perceptions. This bolsters
the conclusion that meta-perceptions are not well differentiated. That
is, people believe that all targets see them in the same way. In sum,
there is a hint of uniqueness in the way Jill sees Jack's personality, but
there is virtually no uniqueness in the way that Jack thinks Jill in particular assesses his personality.

These data on trait perceptions provide some suggestions about
the ways in which social roles may influence social perceptions. First,
perceiver effects in trait perceptions were largest for the applicants'
perceptions of the interviewers in the Kenny and DePaulo (1990) study.
In the same study, the perceiver variance was relatively small for the
interviewers' perceptions of the applicants. This means that the interviewers were much less likely to view all of the applicants similarly
than the applicants were to view the interviewers similarly. This could
have occurred in part because the interviewers were in fact more similar to one another in the way they behaved than were the applicants:
They were told exactly what to ask the applicants, whereas the applicants were not told what to say in response. But, more interestingly,
it could have also occurred in part because the interviewers saw it as
their role to make discriminations among the applicants. Experimental studies in which role is not confounded with other variables could
be designed to address this issue more directly.

It is also interesting in a suggestive way that the three largest estimates of target variance in trait perceptions were from the studies that
involved mixed-sex interactions (Oliver, 1989; Malloy & Janowski,
1992; and Kenny & DePaulo, 1990). Large target variances indicate
that different people agreed in their appraisals of the traits of a given
person. Perhaps this occurred most in the mixed-sex groupings because
perceivers were using gender-based stereotypes.

Affect

As seen in Table 8.3, the variance partitioning for affect is somewhat
similar to that obtained for traits. There is a substantial amount of
perceiver variance for both liking and meta-perceptions. In other words,
there is some consistency in Jill's tendency to like Jack and all the other
people she meets, and there is consistency in Jack's tendency to think
that he is liked by Jill and others, too. As in the trait results, there
is much more perceiver variance for meta-perceptions than for other-
perceptions. Averaging across the five studies, there is 29% more

TABLE 8.3. Variance Partitioning of Affect Studies

Study	Perceiver	Target	Relationship	Error	Rel./err.
Curry & Emerson (1970)					
Week 1					
Liking	.19	.15	—	—	.66
Meta-perception	.42	.10	—	—	.48
Week 8					
Liking	.22	.27	—	—	.50
Meta-perception	.39	.09	—	—	.53
DePaulo et al. (1987)					
Liking	.37	.05	.28	.30	—
Meta-perception	.64	.00	.15	.21	—
Kenny & DePaulo (1990)					
Applicant					
Liking	.25	.12	.32	.30	—
Meta-perception	.71	.01	.04	.24	—
Interviewer					
Liking	.54	.03	.14	.29	—
Meta-perception	.61	.01	.10	.27	—
Oliver (1989)					
Liking	.03	.16	—	—	.81
Meta-perception	.59	.00	—	—	.41
Reno & Kenny (1992)					
Liking	.22	.18	—	—	.59
Meta-perception	.50	.04	—	—	.46
Mean					
Liking	.26	.14	.25	.30	.64
Meta-perception	.55	.04	.10	.24	.47

Note. For Kenny and DePaulo (1990), the "Liking" entries under "Applicant" refer to the interviewers' impressions of the applicants' traits. The "Meta-perception" entries indicate the applicants' beliefs about how they were viewed by others. Similarly, the "Liking" entries under "Interviewer" indicate the applicants' impressions of the interviewers, and the "Meta-perception" entries indicate the interviewers' beliefs about how they were perceived by the applicants. Adapted from Kenny & DePaulo (1993). Copyright 1993 by the American Psychological Association. Adapted by permission.

perceiver variance in meta-perceptions than in liking, and the median level of perceiver variance for meta-perceptions is 59%. So people seem to think that all targets either like or dislike them to the same degree. There is less consistency in the degree to which people like or dislike different targets, a result consistent with the review in Chapter 5.

Does Jack think that Jill likes him because Jill makes everyone feel liked? Probably not. As in the trait results, there is little target variance in meta-perceptions of affect. On average, only 4% of the variance can be attributed to target. This indicates that there is not a consistent tendency for certain targets to be seen as "likers" (people who like everyone) and others as dislikers.

Intuitively, it seems odd that there is so little target variance in meta-perceptions. It is easy to think of people who seem to be stern evaluators of others (e.g., Professor Kingsfield of *The Paper Chase*) and people who seem to be more sympathetic toward others (e.g., Fred Rogers of *Mister Rogers' Neighborhood*). Furthermore, we expect that others would second our nominations of the people in each of these categories. Why, then, are the data at odds with intuition? As always, it is possible that our intuitions are simply wrong (cf. Nisbett & Wilson, 1977). A second possibility is that these meta-perceptions are clouded by self-relevance. Each subject in the studies we reviewed (Kenny & DePaulo, 1993) was asked to indicate not what the target thought of other people, but only what the target thought of the subject himself or herself. So even though Jack, like others, may realize that Jill is no pushover, he may still persist in believing that in her otherwise hard heart, she has a soft spot for him. To test this hypothesis would require subjects to indicate how they think the target views others as well as themselves.

Comparing the trait results in Table 8.2 to the affect results in Table 8.3 indicates that there is about twice as much target variance in the impressions of traits as there is in judgments (not meta-perceptions) of affect. Thus, there is some agreement among targets in the traits they attribute to others. But there is not much agreement about affect—that is, whom they like and whom they dislike (Kenny, 1994). Simply put, affective judgments appear to be more relational than trait judgments. When Jill likes Jack, she seems to see something especially likable about him that most others do not see.

Again, this "specialness" in Jill's liking for Jack and Jack's feeling of being liked by Jill is captured by the relationship component in the variance decomposition. Unfortunately, there are only two studies of affect (both short-term acquaintance studies) in which relationship variance can be separated from error variance. Therefore, all of the conclusions about relationship variance should be regarded as suggestive and in need of replication.

The available studies suggest tentatively that there is some specialness in Jill's liking for Jack. To some (small) degree, Jill does like Jack in a special way that is different from how much she likes others and how much other people like Jack. That is, there is some relationship variance in affect. And there is more of this specialness in Jill's liking for Jack than there is in Jill's perceptions of Jack's personality. That is, there is more relationship variance in affect than in perceptions of traits. This means that there is more differentiation in the degree to which people like particular other people than in the degree to which they view particular others as, say, kind or competent.

Although there is some specialness in Jill's liking for Jack, Jack persists in thinking that everyone likes him, and to about the same degree. That is, there is little relationship variance in meta-perceptions of affect.

Accuracy

It is interesting to learn whether Jack thinks he makes the same impression on Jill that he does on everyone else, or whether he thinks there is something special about the way that Jill views him. In addition, it is at least as interesting to learn whether he is right.

Traits

Table 8.4 presents the accuracy correlations for the studies listed in Table 8.1. Generalized accuracy, again, is the person's ability to predict how others in general view him or her. Clearly, generalized accuracy is fairly high. In the two high acquaintance studies (Malloy & Albright, 1990, and Anderson, 1985), the level of generalized accuracy is very impressive, averaging .58. The study in which the interactions took place in a group (Malloy & Janowski, 1992) shows the highest level of generalized accuracy. The remaining studies involved one-on-one interactions between strangers, and the level of generalized accuracy for these studies, though variable, is always positive. (In two cases, generalized meta-accuracy cannot be computed because there is insufficient target variance in the impressions made by the target on the perceivers. That is, the perceivers do not agree in their impressions of the target; therefore, there is no valid criterion for assessing the accuracy of subjects' estimates of how they are generally viewed by others.) Overall, the level of generalized meta-accuracy for traits is substantial; the median is .58. Therefore, Jack's belief that others generally see him as good-natured and smart is likely to be right.

People's beliefs about how others see them tend to be undifferentiated. Jack, for example, thinks that the many different people he meets all tend to see his personality in about the same way. Because of this, it is unlikely that people are accurate at discerning which targets see

TABLE 8.4. Accuracy Correlations for the Trait Studies

Study	Generalized	Dyadic	Dyadic adjusted
Anderson (1985)	.57	.17	xx
DePaulo et al. (1987)	##	.35	.47
Kenny & DePaulo (1990)			
Applicant	.22	−.07	##
Interviewer	##	.04	##
Malloy & Albright (1990)	.59	.10	xx
Malloy & Janowski (1992)	.73	.10	.14
Oliver (1989)	.69	.19	xx
Reno & Kenny (1992)	.26	.16	xx
Mean	.51	.13	

Note. ## = less than 5% of the variance; correlation not computed. xx = single replication; adjustment not possible. Adapted from Kenny and DePaulo (1993). Copyright 1993 by the American Psychological Association. Adapted by permission.

them as especially high on a trait and which targets see them as low. This is what dyadic accuracy measures: people's understanding of how they are uniquely viewed by particular other people.

Although seven of the eight dyadic-accuracy correlations are positive (see Table 8.4), they are all quite weak. The largest correlation is for DePaulo, Kenny, Hoover, Webb, and Oliver (1987). Because these correlations contain error variance, they may be attenuated as a result of measurement error. However, the disattenuated correlations (dyadic adjusted) are not much larger. Therefore, people seem to have just a tiny glimmer of insight into how they are uniquely viewed by particular other people.

Affect

It has been shown that people are accurate at knowing how others generally view their personalities. Are they also accurate at knowing how much others generally like them? That is, do they know whether they are popular? Table 8.5 shows the accuracy correlations for affect. For all five studies, generalized accuracy is positive; for some of them, it is substantial. These affect correlations are not quite as high as the trait correlations; probably because there is more target variance in the trait studies than in the affect studies. Perceivers seem to agree with one another more when evaluating a particular person's personality than when indicating how much they like that person. (That

TABLE 8.5. Accuracy Correlations for the Affect Studies

Study	Generalized	Dyadic	Dyadic adjusted
Curry & Emerson (1970)			
Week 1	.40	.35	xx
Week 8	.21	.43	xx
DePaulo et al. (1987)	##	.20	.17
Kenny & DePaulo (1990)			
Applicant	.47	−.17	##
Interviewer	##	−.04	##
Oliver (1989)	1.00	.37	xx
Reno & Kenny (1992)	.29	.09	xx
Mean	.47	.18	

Note. ## = less than 5% of the variance; correlation not computed. xx = single replication; adjustment not possible. Adapted from Kenny and DePaulo (1993). Copyright 1993 by the American Psychological Association. Adapted by permission.

is, there is more target variance in perceptions of traits than in perceptions of affect.) Therefore, it is probably easier for the persons being evaluated to discern how they are generally viewed on, say, sociability and intelligence than to determine how much they are generally liked.

Dyadic accuracy for affect indicates whether people know which particular other people especially like them. The results for relationship effects, reviewed above, suggest that there is some differentiation in the degree to which other people like a particular person. Jill's liking for Jack, for example, is to some extent unique to Jack. Furthermore, there may be a bit more differentiation in these perceptions of liking than there is for perceptions of traits. Therefore, it should be easier for people to know who uniquely likes them than it is for them to know who sees them as especially good-natured or intelligent. Table 8.5 shows the dyadic-accuracy correlations for affect. These correlations are positive for all except the Kenny and DePaulo (1990) study. Although they are only small or moderate in magnitude, they are, as expected, somewhat larger than the analogous dyadic correlations for traits.

Correlates of the Perceiver Effect in Meta-Perceptions

As shown in Tables 8.2 and 8.3, people believe that they make either consistently good or bad impressions on others. Although there is some degree of validity in these perceptions, this perceived consistency may also reflect some underlying psychological disposition. For example, are people who are especially dependent on the approval of others particularly likely to think that others generally think well of them? Data relevant to this hypothesis are available from the studies we reviewed (Kenny & DePaulo, 1993) in which individual differences were assessed. Considered are only those individual-difference variables measured in two or more studies—private and public self-consciousness, social anxiety, self-monitoring, and need for social approval (see Table 8.6). The correlations between these five variables and the perceiver

TABLE 8.6. Correlations of Individual-Difference Variables with the Perceiver Effect in Meta-Perceptions

Variable	Trait	Affect
Private self-consciousness		
DePaulo et al. (1987)	−.09	−.09
Malloy & Albright (1990)	.01	##
Malloy & Janowski (1992)	.12	##
Reno & Kenny (1992)	−.04	−.12
Public self-consciousness		
DePaulo et al. (1987)	−.08	.00
Malloy & Albright (1990)	.07	##
Malloy & Janowski (1992)	−.09	##
Reno & Kenny (1992)	.27	.24
Social anxiety		
DePaulo et al. (1987)	−.56	−.49
Malloy & Albright (1990)	−.24	##
Malloy & Janowski (1992)	−.22	##
Reno & Kenny (1992)	.06	−.14
Need for social approval		
DePaulo et al. (1987)	.14	.39
Oliver (1989)	.54	.52
Self-monitoring		
DePaulo et al. (1987)	.24	.11
Malloy & Albright (1990)	−.04	##
Malloy & Janowski (1992)	−.12	##
Oliver (1989)	−.31	−.43

Note. ## = less than 5% of the variance; correlation not computed. Adapted from Kenny and DePaulo (1993). Copyright 1993 by the American Psychological Association. Adapted by permission.

effect in meta-perceptions (how people think they are generally viewed by others) are shown in Table 8.6.

The first two variables examined are private and public self-consciousness (Fenigstein, Scheier, & Buss, 1975); private self-consciousness is clearly not related to meta-perceptions, and public self-consciousness is correlated with meta-perceptions only in the Reno and Kenny (1992) study. Self-monitoring effects are weak except for the Oliver (1989) study. For social anxiety, five of the six correlations are negative, and they are particularly strong in the DePaulo et al. (1987) study. Socially anxious people, then, generally think that they convey unflattering impressions of themselves to others. This finding has also been reported in studies of social anxiety using different methodologies (e.g., Crozier, 1979; Jones & Briggs, 1984; Teglasi & Hoffman, 1982).

The correlations for social approval are always positive; thus, people who are high in need for approval say that they generally make positive impressions on others.[2] It can be concluded either that meta-perceptions are subject to response set or that this supports the measure's validity. Note that the correlations in the Oliver (1989) study may be stronger because subjects were selected to be in the top and bottom quartiles of need for social approval.

The results in Table 8.6 suggest that a need for social approval does consistently predict meta-perceptions, but there are just two studies for this variable. Social anxiety does strongly predict meta-perceptions. The other personality variables do not show a consistent pattern.

Whether there is any validity to these beliefs can be addressed by correlating subjects' scores on social anxiety and need for approval with the impressions that others generally formed of them (i.e., target effect in other-perceptions). (In DePaulo et al., 1987, subjects did not make consistent impressions on their partners; therefore, the question of the relationship of that variance to individual differences cannot be assessed.) For need for approval, there are two relevant correlations, both from the Oliver (1989) study. Subjects high in need for approval were in fact generally liked more by others (the correlation is .34), and they were also seen as more active (dominant, confident, outgoing, and imaginative; the average correlation is .31). There are also two estimates for social anxiety, and they too are in the expected direction, both being −.32. Socially anxious people, who think they make poor impressions on others, were in fact evaluated harshly by the other subjects in the Malloy and Janowski (1992) and the Malloy and Albright (1990) studies.

In sum, then, the data suggest that there is some validity to different meta-perceptions of people who vary in need for approval and social anxiety. Approval-dependent people do seem to make better impressions on others, just as they believe they do; and socially anxious people do seem to make the negative impressions that they fear. Furthermore, this occurs even during brief interactions with strangers.

As is discussed later in this chapter, these data provide suggestive evidence for the argument that when people attain accuracy at finding out how others view them, they can do so even without paying much attention to the ways in which those people are reacting to them. Socially anxious people bring with them to their social interactions an expectation that they will not make a very good impression. Often, others really do take a dim view of them. If socially anxious people simply stand by their predictions, without bothering to check their validity against the data of the ongoing interaction, they are often right about how they are viewed by others. They can be right not because they have observed and understood the reactions of others, but because they understand themselves.

Self-Perception and Meta-Perception

In the review of the individual-difference results above, it has been suggested that people may simply assume that others see them the way they see themselves. It has been shown, for example, that people who describe themselves as evaluatively dependent expect to be viewed positively by others, and that others generally do view them positively. However, this relationship between the ways that people view themselves and the ways they believe they are viewed by others can be assessed more directly by simply correlating self-perceptions with meta-perceptions.

As usual, this relationship can be evaluated in two different ways. First, it can be asked whether people who generally rate themselves positively believe that they are generally viewed positively by others. When subjects in a study only state their general self-perceptions (as in Anderson, 1985, Malloy & Albright, 1990; Malloy & Janowski, 1992; and Reno & Kenny, 1992), this correlation between self-perceptions and perceiver effects in meta-perceptions is the only kind that can be computed. When instead, for *each* of their interactions, subjects rate themselves and also indicate the impressions they thought they made on their partners (as in Kenny & DePaulo, 1990, and Oliver, 1989), self-perceptions can be correlated with both the perceiver and relationship effects in meta-perceptions. The correlations with relationship effects indicate whether people who rate themselves differently during different interactions also think that they are rated

TABLE 8.7. Self- and Meta-Perception Correlations

Study	Generalized	Dyadic	Dyadic adjusted
Kenny & DePaulo (1990)			
Trait			
Applicant	.99	.49	.29
Interviewer	.98	.66	##
Affect			
Applicant	.96	.66	##
Interviewer	.97	.70	##
Oliver (1989)			
Trait	.97	.64	xx
Affect	1.00	.47	xx
Anderson (1985)	.51	—	—
Malloy & Albright (1990)	.66	—	—
Malloy & Janowski (1992)	1.00	—	—
Reno & Kenny (1992)			
Trait	.75	—	—
Affect	.80	—	—
Mean	.87	.60	

Note. ## = less than 5% of the variance; correlation not computed. xx = single replication; adjustment not possible. — = self-perceptions not measured for each target. Adapted from Kenny and DePaulo (1993). Copyright 1993 by the American Psychological Association. Adapted by permission.

differently by others during those different interactions. Table 8.7 shows the correlations between self-perceptions and meta-perceptions for all six of these studies.

First considered is the generalized level. As seen in Table 8.7, there is a strong correlation between how subjects viewed themselves and how they thought others saw them. The "weakest" correlation is .51. The two residential studies, Anderson (1985) and Malloy and Albright (1990), show the lowest correlations. In these two studies, the self-perception was a general perception, not a perception of the self in the context of a study. At the dyadic level, there are also impressive correlations between self- and meta-perception. So if people see themselves as acting differently with different people, they think that the different targets see them differently too.

The very large magnitude of the correlations between self-perceptions and other-perceptions at both the generalized and dyadic levels raises the question of whether the correlations are as big as they are because of shared method variance. Both self-perceptions and meta-perceptions are self-report measures involving analogous rating scales. However, this argument is weakened by the fact that every correlation in Table 8.7, with only one exception (affect for the Oliver study), is greater than the corresponding correlation between the perceiver effect in other-perception and self-perception. If shared method variance caused the correlations in Table 8.7 between self-perception and meta-perception, then shared method variance should produce equally large correlations between self-perception and other-perception. Further evidence for the discriminant validity of self-perceptions and meta-perceptions comes from studies in which the mean level of subjects' self-perceptions differs from the mean level of their meta-perceptions. For example, Campbell and Fehr (1990) documented such differences between self-perceptions and meta-perceptions, and also showed that those discrepancies varied systematically with subjects' self-esteem. There is also evidence that self-perceptions and meta-perceptions are differentially affected by evaluative feedback (Wyer, Henninger, & Wolfson, 1975).

Reciprocity and Assumed Reciprocity: Attaining Accuracy by Assuming Reciprocity

People can be accurate in their assessments of how others view them without paying much attention to the way others are actually reacting to them if they base their assessments on their perceptions of themselves (e.g., socially anxious people think they make bad impressions) and those perceptions are true. There is another way in which people can attain accuracy without attending to feedback: They may assume that there is reciprocity in people's liking for each other and in their evaluation of each other's traits. If Jack sees Jill as good-natured, he may just assume that Jill also sees him as good-natured. He may do so without even bothering to look to Jill to see whether she seems to be regarding him as good-natured. If Jack's theory is right — if perceptions of traits really are reciprocated — then his belief that Jill sees him as good-natured is also right. Jack's meta-perceptions are accurate, but not (necessarily) because he is paying attention to feedback from others.

To evaluate the hypothesis that people may attain accuracy by assuming reciprocity (Kenny & Albright, 1987), it must be determined whether people really do assume reciprocity and whether reciprocity does in fact exist. In Chapter 6, in Table 6.6, correlations for the actual reciprocity of impressions (if Jack sees Jill as sociable, does Jill see Jack as sociable?) and the perceived reciprocity between meta-perception and the impression (if Jack sees Jill as sociable, does he think that Jill sees him as sociable?) have been presented. For traits, with hardly any exception, neither type of reciprocity is very strong; perceptions of reciprocity are stronger than actual reciprocity in most cases, but the levels of assumed reciprocity are not high. For affect, both types of reciprocity are higher than the corresponding reciprocities for traits. Furthermore, in most cases people assume more reciprocity of liking — sometimes much more — than actually exists; assumed reciprocity of liking is substantial for virtually every study. (See Table 6.6 and Chapter 6 for further details.)

When are people accurate in their beliefs about who likes them? These data suggest that they are accurate when their assumption of reciprocity is in fact true. People generally assume that people they like also like them in return. That assumption does not vary much from person to person or from study to study. What does matter, then, in determining whether people's meta-perceptions are accurate is whether reciprocity of liking really does exist. If people believe that their liking is reciprocated, and it really is, then their beliefs about who does and does not like them will be correct.

Theoretical Integration

Basis of Meta-Perceptions: Self-Perceptions, Not Feedback from Others

How do people determine how others view them? The most obvious answer to this question — that people observe others' reactions to their behavior and base their meta-perceptions on that feedback — is the least likely to be correct. Instead, it may be that people's beliefs about how others view them are based primarily on their perceptions of themselves.

Several lines of evidence support the self-perception explanation. First, in an absolute sense, the amount of variance accounted for by perceiver effects in meta-perception is quite high. That is, there is a strong tendency for people to think that they make consistent impressions on the various targets with whom they interact. In fact, however, different targets often form very different impressions of them, especially in regard to how much they like them.

Second, perceiver effects are stronger for meta-perceptions than for other-perceptions. This provides discriminant validity for the importance of perceiver effects in meta-perceptions, in that it indicates that not all perceiver effects are equally strong. It is when people are estimating the impressions they convey to different target persons that they are especially likely to make consistent judgments. They are not nearly as consistent when they attribute a particular trait or affect to a variety of target persons.

Third, the amount of relationship variance in meta-perceptions is typically small in an absolute sense, and it is usually smaller than the amount of relationship variance in other-perceptions. This means that people tend not to think that they are seen in unique ways by particular other people, as they might if they were noticing variations in the ways that different targets react to them. Sometimes they do see some uniqueness, but it is usually not as much uniqueness as they ascribe to particular other people in attributing traits or affects to them.

Fourth, generalized meta-accuracy is always greater than dyadic meta-accuracy (for all comparisons in which both scores are available) for traits, and for affect it is greater in four of five comparisons. This indicates that people's impressions of how they are generally viewed by others are more accurate than their differential impressions of how they are uniquely viewed by particular others. Again, if people were attuned to the feedback provided by targets during ongoing social interactions, they might attain higher levels of dyadic accuracy.

Finally, and perhaps most compelling, the relationships between self-perceptions and meta-perceptions are quite high. As seen in Table 8.7, there is strong correspondence between how people see themselves and how they think that others see them.

Before the implications of these results for theory are considered, a general model of meta-perception is displayed in Figure 8.1. Jack has general views about what kind of person he is. This view affects how he behaves with others (path *a*) and how he interprets his behavior with others (path *b*). Jack's behavior affects how Jill reacts to Jack[3] (path *c*) and Jack's self-evaluation (path *d*). Jack's meta-perception of

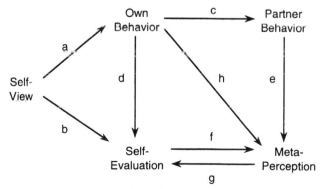

FIGURE 8.1. Model of the formation of meta-perception.

how Jill sees him is affected by Jill's behavior (path *e*), his behavior (path *h*), and his self-evaluation (path *f*). Finally, Jack's self-evaluation (and eventually his self-concept) may be affected by his meta-perception (path *g*).

In the symbolic-interactionist or "naive" model, the causation goes from one's own behavior to the partner's behavior (path *c*), from the partner's behavior to meta-perception (path *e*), and from meta-perception to self-evaluation (path *g*). This variant of the model presented in Figure 8.1 is presented in the top of Figure 8.2.

All of the data reviewed so far are more consistent with a self-perception explanation of meta-perceptions than with a feedback explanation. The self-perception explanation can now be articulated further. Three different versions are considered, and the models (which are simpler variants of the model in Figure 8.1) are also presented in Figure 8.2.

The simplest of these is the "self-theory" version. According to this version, people have strongly held theories about their own personalities. When interacting with others, they believe that their own personalities as they see them are immediately apparent to others, even during relatively brief interactions with total strangers (path *b*). People not only can disregard their partners' behavior in determining how their partners view them; they can also disregard their own behavior (paths *c* and *d* are zero).

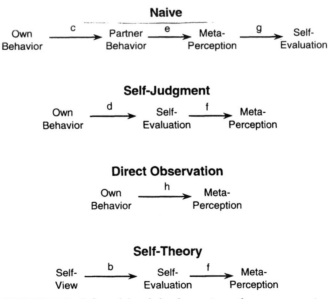

FIGURE 8.2. Submodels of the formation of meta-perception.

The other two versions assume that people do observe their own behaviors when trying to determine how others view them. In one version, the "self-judgment" version (Felson, 1992), people observe their own behavior, make a judgment or self-perception about that behavior (path d), and then assume that others see that behavior the same way they do (path f). The process begins with the observation of one's own behavior, which leads to a self-perception, which then leads to a meta-perception. Jack observes himself frolicking merrily on the hill, judges himself to be quite a good-natured chap, and assumes that Jill thinks so too.

In the third version, the "direct-observation" version, perception of one's own behavior leads directly to a meta-perception (path h). People observe their own behavior in an attempt to determine what impressions other people may be forming of them on the basis of that behavior. In this version, these observations do not necessarily change self-views. Jack observes himself frolicking merrily and thinks that Jill sees him as good-natured.

Many of the results described in this chapter are consistent with the view that people simply assume that their personalities are immediately apparent to others—the self-theory version. The large perceiver variances in meta-perceptions, indicating that people think that different partners all tend to view them in the same way, follow easily from this formulation. So does the small degree of relationship effects (or specialness) in meta-perceptions. The high degree of generalized accuracy that people attain can also be accommodated. If people's theories about themselves are correct, then their beliefs about how others generally view them are also correct. Finally, the strong correlations between self-perceptions and meta-perceptions are also very much in accord with the view that people simply assume that others see them as they already see themselves.

Most troubling to the self-theory version is the fact that people do achieve a measure of dyadic accuracy. If it were true that they really pay no attention at all to their own or to their partners' behaviors, then they could not discern any real differences in the ways that different partners view them.

The non-negligible levels of dyadic accuracy could be troubling to all of the versions of the self-perception perspective if dyadic accuracy could be attained only by attending to feedback from one's interaction partners. However, it is possible for people to learn about differences in how different partners are viewing them simply by observing their own behavior. For if people's behavior differs with partners who view them differently, then they can learn about those varying views of themselves simply by examining their own behavior.

When people interact with different people one at a time, then their behavior really differs from partner to partner. However, when people interact with all of their partners at the same time, though each partner's reaction may differ, their own behavior remains the same. All of their partners have the same information about them. It follows from this analysis that if dyadic accuracy is based on observations of one's own behavior, it should be higher in studies in which people interact one-on-one (and their behavior therefore does vary from partner to partner) than in studies in which people interact in groups. Three of the trait studies involved one-on-one interactions: DePaulo et al. (1987), Oliver (1989), and Reno and Kenny (1992). Although none of these studies show impressively high levels of dyadic meta-accuracy, there is heightened meta-accuracy relative to the levels in the other studies. Interestingly, the Reno and Kenny (1992) study, which included ratings that may have been among the most behavioral (e.g., amount of information conveyed), shows the narrowest gap between generalized and dyadic accuracy. These kinds of issues could be addressed more compellingly by experiments in which subjects are randomly assigned to group versus dyadic interactions, and make meta-perceptions along dimensions known to vary in visibility.

The finding that people do achieve some meta-accuracy, then, is consistent with both the self-judgment and the direct-observation versions, for in both versions, people observe their own behavior. That behavior can reveal to them differences in the ways they are responding to partners who have different views of them. One line of evidence that is especially supportive of the self-judgment version is the set of strong correlations between self-perceptions and meta-perceptions. The self-judgment perspective insists that people observe their own behavior, make self-perceptions, and then assume that others view them as they view themselves. If this is really how people figure out how others view them, then the correlations between self-perceptions and meta-perceptions have to be high. Furthermore, any evidence that self-perceptions are not just correlated with meta-perceptions, but precede them temporally, would also suit the self-judgment perspective well. This evidence is reviewed in the next section.

The direct-observation version of self-perception makes no such assumptions about the relationship between self-perceptions and other-perceptions. Instead, it argues that people simply observe their own behavior and try to determine what impressions their partners are likely to form of them on the basis of that behavior. This version credits people with a bit of perspective taking that the self-judgment version denies. Any evidence, then, that people sometimes do think that others view their behavior differently than they do is evidence that favors the direct-observation perspective.

Several studies do provide just such data. In a study by Wyer et al. (1975), women who received performance feedback in front of an observer believed that the feedback would affect the observer's view of them, but it did not affect their own self-views. Similarly, Felson (1992) found that subjects' performance directly affected the subjects' beliefs about how others viewed them, even when their own self-perceptions had been statistically controlled. Finally, Swann and Hill (1982) showed that when people's self-views were challenged, they worked to reaffirm them by behaving in a particularly self congruent manner. This opportunity to refute the feedback through behavior helped the subjects to maintain their self-views. Importantly, they stood by their self-views even when they believed that their partners remained unconvinced by their self-affirming efforts.

Among the three versions of the self-perception perspective, the direct-observation model may have a bit of an edge. However, probably each version is used at times, and each can be a road to accuracy.

Self-Perceptions to Meta-Perceptions or Vice Versa?

The causal direction being assumed is from self-perception to meta-perception. So in Figure 8.1, path f is assumed to exist, and path g is assumed to be small. This is the opposite of what the symbolic interactionists suggest. They argue that self-perceptions are products of the beliefs about how the self is viewed by significant others; they are the reflections that the self sees in other people's eyes. There are several reasons to conclude that self-perceptions are primary.

First, there are real differences in how different people view the same person. This is known from the data from the eight studies we reviewed (Kenny & DePaulo, 1993): Generally different partners did indeed form different impressions of any given subject. This was especially so for how much they liked the subject. Yet subjects were almost completely oblivious to these differences; they thought they made essentially the same impression on all of their partners.

The second source of evidence suggesting a chain of causality from self-perception to meta-perception rather than vice versa consists of the data on individual differences. From study to study, socially anxious individuals thought that others looked askance at them. In contrast, subjects high in need for approval thought consistently that others looked favorably upon them. Subjects brought their social anxiety levels and their approval needs with them to the studies in which they participated; they did not acquire those self-concepts from the ways they thought they were viewed by their partners during the study. Yet those self-qualities seemed to drive their perceptions of how others were reacting to them.

Similarly, in their study of the relationship between self-esteem and perceptions of popularity, Bohrnstedt and Felson (1983) showed that children who liked themselves assumed that other children also liked them. Models in which self-esteem affected meta-perceptions of popularity fit the data better than those in which the reverse or reciprocal effects were estimated.

The individual-difference results reported in this chapter are consistent with data reported by Felson (1981) in his study of high school football players. Players' self-ratings on ambiguous attributes such as "football sense" and "mental toughness" correlated near zero with the coaches' ratings of them. Therefore, the players were not discerning their coaches' actual assessments of them and internalizing those appraisals; their self-ratings were correlated with their own self-confidence, as rated both by themselves and by their coaches. What the data suggest, as Felson notes, is that self-concept is not constructed impartially from the data available in social life; instead, "persons see either what they expect or want to see" (p. 68).

Other research also underscores the strength of self-conceptions in shaping social interactions, social perceptions, and the views that others come to hold about targets. Most notably, Swann (e.g., 1984, 1990; Swann & Hill, 1982) has amassed a wealth of data indicating that people work to confirm their self-views—usually successfully. For example, in one study, subjects with certain or uncertain self-concepts interacted with partners with certain or uncertain views of the subjects that were inconsistent with the subjects' self-views (Swann & Ely, 1984). Over the course of successive interactions, the subjects—particularly those who held their self-views with certainty—came to be viewed by their partners in the way that they viewed themselves. That is, the partners adopted the subjects' views of themselves, rather than vice versa. The only exception to this pattern occurred when the partners were confident about their views of subjects who were unsure of their own self-concepts.

What Are Subjects Doing with the Available Feedback from Their Interaction Partners?

If the views that people think others have of them are derived from observing their own behavior and from their own views of themselves, then are people paying any attention at all to the texture of their partners' behavior? It seems plausible that they are. Evidence comes from the other-perception data: Perceiver variances are smaller for other-perceptions than they are for meta-perceptions, and relationship effects are larger. This suggests that people do see differences among the various other people in their social worlds. Moreover, the differences that they see are not idiosyncratic. Other people concur, at least somewhat, in their assessments of a given target's traits, and they even show a bit of agreement in their appraisals of the target's likability (as indicated by the nontrivial target effects in other-perceptions). So when they are asked to assess qualities of their partners, people seem able to attend to the available data and make an evaluation for which there is consensual validation. What they seem unable to assess in a differentiated way are the variations in how these different partners see the people themselves.

There are many reasons for this insensitivity. First, because of people's reluctance to evaluate one another explicitly, the quality of the available data is poor. Second, people are personally invested in their self-concepts (e.g., Swann, 1990), and therefore they are also invested in the perceptions that others have of them. This investment far outstrips any investments that they might have in their perceptions of other people. That is, they care about how others view them far more than they care how they view others. Third, in reading others' reactions, people often see what they expect to see. These expectations in turn came from many sources, including people's self-concepts, their knowledge of the kinds of impressions they may be *trying* to convey, and their minitheories about the workings of social life (such as the expectation that liking is reciprocated).

Limitations and Qualifications

Do Self-Perceptions Always Come First?

Arguing that self-perceptions drive meta-perceptions rather than vice versa does not mean that people's beliefs about how others view them never affect their self-views. If, repeatedly, a person is the last to be chosen when captains pick teams, and the only one without a date to the ball, it will be difficult for the person not to form the impression that others find him or her inept or unlovable, and perhaps more difficult still to remain unscathed by this impression. Over the long run, then, the glare of others' mirrors may simply be too overpowering to ignore. The support of intimates who view the person as he or she views himself or herself can help deflect that glare; but when intimates disagree with self-views, too, then the mirror wins again, perhaps even more triumphantly (Swann & Predmore, 1985).

Even in short-lived interactions with strangers, there are times when meta-perceptions change self-perceptions. This may occur when people are outcome-dependent on their interaction partners (e.g., when they are powerful, influential, or attractive people). It may occur when others are evaluating targets on dimensions along which the targets' standing is a matter of great concern but little certainty. And it may also occur during transitions to new and unfamiliar life situations, such as going away to college or beginning one's first job.

Symbolic interactionism is a theory of development as well as a theory of social interaction, and its developmental predictions may fare better than the other predictions in this chapter (Rosenberg, 1986). Over the course of development, children may indeed construct their self-concepts at least in part from their beliefs about how they are viewed by others. Moreover, parents may be more willing than peers or strangers to provide negative feedback to their children. There is some suggestive evidence that is consistent with this hypothesized developmental process (Felson, 1989; Rosengren, 1961). The Felson study has shown, using longitudinal data, that appraisals of children by their parents affect children's subsequent meta-perceptions. But this important study has also shown that children think that both parents view them in the same way—a result consistent with the finding of large amounts of perceiver variance in meta-perceptions.

A developmental perspective may also help to explain why adults sometimes seem so oblivious to the feedback available to them in ongoing social interactions. Perhaps they pay so little attention to that feedback in the present because they paid so much attention to it in the past. As children, perhaps they did look into other people's eyes to see inside their own psyches. Many thousands of looks later, they may have come to develop quite stable self-concepts. They may feel, as adults, that it is no longer necessary to take a fresh look into others' eyes during each interaction. They have looked there often before, and know what to expect.

A similar process may occur during the development of a close relationship (see also Swann & Predmore, 1985). At first, Jack cannot stop looking into Jill's eyes. Eventually, though, he thinks he knows what he will see there, and his eyes will rest elsewhere. Sometimes Jill's reaction to Jack is not what Jack would have expected, but he will not know that, because he is not paying much attention. If this sad sequence does in fact occur, one counterintuitive implication may be that dyadic meta-accuracy does not necessarily improve over time as relationships progress.

How Far Will the Results Generalize?

It may be tempting to conclude that the results apply more to short-term interactions than to long-term ones. The argument would be that people rely primarily on their self-perceptions during brief interactions because there is not much else to go by. Yet a recent review has indicated that even very thin slices of expressive behavior (i.e., ones lasting less than 5 minutes) can be surprisingly informative (Ambady & Rosenthal, 1992).

Similarly, an intuitively appealing prediction would be that the results do not generalize to people in long-term intimate relationships. But as just argued in the preceding section, when relationships develop, partners may actually become *less* attuned to each other's feedback during ongoing social interactions, because they think they already know what that feedback will be.

Another limitation of the studies reviewed is that the subjects in all of them were college undergraduates. Furthermore, the students always rated one another on positive traits. Perhaps work with other populations and other kinds of ratings will point to important qualifications of the conclusions. It is also possible that systematic manipulations of aspects of the social context and of subjects' social interaction goals will add further qualifications. But extensions of this work will serve to underscore some of the more robust findings. There are already hints that this will be so. For example, it has been found that people are very good at understanding how they are generally viewed by others, but that they are much less adept at discerning how they are uniquely viewed by particular others. In a series of studies of populations other than college students, Felson (1980, 1981, 1989) has reported very similar effects.

Most of the results presented in this chapter have been replicated in a study done in Israel (Shechtman & Kenny, in press). That study, also using college students, shows that the conclusions in this chapter are not as limited as they might appear.

The purpose is not to deny the possible limitations of the results, but to encourage open-minded investigations of them. The major limitations of the studies that have been reviewed are that none of them (1) measured the behaviors of either interactant or (2) experimentally manipulated the key constructs, such as partner feedback. The behavior of the person who makes the meta-perception should better predict that person's meta-perceptions than the feedback behavior of that person's interaction partner. Studies with such measurements and manipulations are difficult and time-consuming, but they are necessary to illuminate the exact causal sequence.

Conclusion

How do people know how others view them? The first conclusion is a counterintuitive one: People rely very little on feedback from others.

Instead, they directly observe their own behavior, and infer from it what others think of them. This conclusion is based on evidence showing that people think that the impressions they make on different people are more consistent than they are in fact; that people are better at discerning what other people generally think of them than in deciphering the unique ways that particular other people view them; and, finally, that people's reports of how they think others view them are highly correlated with how they view themselves.

The second and related conclusion may be a controversial one: Symbolic interactionists have the direction of causality exactly wrong, at least for adults. People's self-perceptions do not come from their beliefs about how others view them (meta-perceptions); instead, meta-perceptions follow directly from self-perceptions. When people observe their own behavior to try to discern what others think of them, their theories about themselves and about social life are important in determining what they see. To the extent that these theories are correct, then their understandings of how others generally view them are also correct.

If people were to rely *only* on their self-concepts and their theories to interpret the data of their behavior and others' reactions to that behavior, then the best they could achieve would be generalized accuracy. People could never figure out how they are differentially viewed by particular others. But in fact, people are not totally oblivious to the behavior of specific other people. They notice things about them that others notice, too. The third and final conclusion is that people do achieve some small degree of dyadic accuracy in their perceptions of how specific others view them. Occasionally, then, people do look to others for feedback, and thereby catch a glimpse of how those others really do see them.

This chapter has tied together several empirical studies. It very convincingly shows that people think that they make consistent impressions on their partners when in fact they do not, at least not to the extent that they think they do. Meta-perceptions are partially accurate, but it seems that the accuracy in meta-perceptions is attained through inference and not from feedback. It has been shown that self-perception is closely tied to meta-perception. The next chapter considers the topic of self-perception.

Notes

1. Perceiver accuracy is not considered, because there is typically little or no target variance in meta-perceptions.

2. The correlation between social anxiety and need for social approval is zero in the DePaulo et al. (1987) study.

3. It is possible that the partner's behavior may influence one's own behavior, but to make the analysis manageable, this effect is ignored.

Chapter 9

SELF-PERCEPTION

The perception of others is very closely tied to self-perception. People are very much concerned about whether they are similar to others on some traits (e.g., emotional stability), or better than others on other traits (e.g., intelligence). As reviewed in Chapter 8, it appears that meta-perception is largely guided by self-perception. This chapter elaborates the links between other-perception and self-perception.

The chapter begins with a discussion of the major social psychological theories about self-perception. Next discussed is whether people engage in self-enhancement: To what extent do people view themselves more favorably than they view others?

The middle part of the chapter concerns assumed similarity: Do people see others as they see themselves? First, there is a discussion of the extent to which there is assumed similarity. The next question is whether the perceiver effect has more influence in other-perception than in self-perception. A discussion of the effect of acquaintance on assumed similarity follows.

The third section of this chapter concerns self–other agreement. The first question considered is the *level* of self–other agreement. The second question concerns whether peers agree more with each other than they do with the self. The third question concerns whether self-ratings or peer ratings are more accurate. The fourth question concerns the conditions under which there is more or less self–other agreement. The fifth and final question concerns the social-psychological processes that explain self–other agreement. So the first three questions about self–other agreement concern the level of self–other agreement; the fourth concerns moderators; and the fifth concerns the theoretical explanation of the phenomenon.

In the final section, the variability of self-ratings and other-ratings is compared.

Theories of Self-Perception

The topic of self is one of the oldest in psychology (William James, one of the first psychologists, wrote extensively on it), and a consideration of the different ways social scientists have treated it should be helpful. In connection with each theory, individual differences are also discussed: To what extent do some people conform more to the theoretical perspective than do others? Table 9.1 presents a summary of the theories and their associated individual differences.

One view of self-perception, initially proposed by the social psychologist Daryl Bem (1967), is that it is little different from other-perception. Other-perception results from behavioral observation; that is, people observe others and infer that those others have certain personalities. Self-perception, according to Bem, also results from the observation of behavior. (See Chapter 8.) From this perspective, self-perception is not based on privileged access. That is, if I am judging how friendly I am, I look at my behavior to see how friendly I am. I do not look inside myself at my motives and intentions to ascertain my friendliness. So I evaluate my friendliness in the same way as I would evaluate another person's friendliness.

Bem's view of self-perception may be more true of people who do not introspect and wonder very much about what types of persons they are. Fenigstein, Scheier, and Buss (1975) have proposed that people differ in how privately self-conscious they are. "Private self-consciousness" refers to introspection and self-contemplation, whereas "public self-consciousness" refers to a fear of negative evaluations from others. People who are more privately self-conscious should have a better idea of what types of persons they are, and should be less likely to use the process proposed by Bem.

A second view is that self-perception is largely guided by the motive of "self-enhancement." People try to foster a positive image of themselves; therefore, they deny or downplay their negative characteristics and emphasize their positive ones. As the term suggests, people en-

TABLE 9.1. Theories of Self

Theory name	Individual-difference variable
Self-perception	Private self-consciousness
Self-enhancement	Depression, self-esteem
Self-presentation	Self-monitoring, need for social approval
Symbolic interactionism versus self-verification	Certainty

gage in self-enhancement in order to make themselves feel better. If the goal were to create a favorable impression on *others,* then it would be called "self-presentation" (which is discussed later in this section). Although self-enhancement is a form of biased information processing, it is a normal process. That is, some degree of self-enhancement is typically found in self-ratings. In fact, Taylor and Brown (1988) have argued that self-enhancement is necessary for mental health, and they have claimed that normal, healthy adults engage in it regularly.

Although clearly self-enhancement is a general motive, some people self-enhance more than others. Several individual-difference variables have been shown to affect the degree of self-enhancement. The most extensively studied variable has been depression (Alloy & Abramson, 1988; Lewinsohn, Mischel, Chaplin, & Barton, 1980). Not surprisingly, depressives (as well as those low in self-esteem) self-enhance less than nondepressives do. This fact has led some to argue that depressives are more accurate person perceivers than nondepressives; this hypothesis, called "depressive realism," is disputed by some (e.g., Campbell & Fehr, 1990).

The third view, "self-presentation," is that people present images of themselves to others, much in the same way that political consultants create images of political candidates in television commercials. This view was espoused by the sociologist Erving Goffman (1959). Borrowing a line from Shakespeare, Goffman viewed social life as a stage and people as actors giving performances to an audience. If the audience or role changes, so does a person's behavior. In this view, people are social chameleons who change their behavior to please different audiences.

Mark Snyder (1974) has proposed that some people self-present more than others, and has called such people "high self-monitors." Others, called "low self-monitors," tend not to tailor their behavior to match audience expectations. Another measure of self-presentational tendencies is the need for social approval, usually called "social desirability." This variable represents the motive to be liked and approved by others. Presumably, people who are high on the need for social approval engage in self-presentation more often than those who are low on the need for social approval. Interestingly, the correlation between Snyder's self-monitoring scale and the Crowne and Marlowe (1960) scale of social desirability is negative (Oliver, 1989). It is possible that the correlation is negative because self-monitoring may not be a desirable skill; that is, it may be socially desirable to say that one does not self-present.

A fourth and final view is a combination of clinical and sociological views. In this perspective, the self-concept is learned during childhood: The child incorporates the view that parents have of the child. So if parents say to the child, "You stupid idiot, why do you do these things?", the child sees himself or herself as a "stupid idiot." Sociologists, beginning with the ground-breaking efforts of George Herbert Mead (1925, 1934) and Cooley (1902), have developed the theory of "symbolic interactionism" (see Chapter 8). People incorporate the view that significant others have of them. The self, something that we think of as private and personal, is a social creation. Clinical psychologists such as Carl Rogers and Harry Stack Sullivan have espoused a similar view: They focus on people who have negative self-perceptions, and believe that these self-images arose from negative interactions with parents.

Symbolic interactionism is similar to the self-presentation view in that the person is influenced by others. But it differs from self-presentation in that the person actually incorporates the view that others have of him or her. According to symbolic interactionists, people see themselves as others see them.

That people adopt the views that others have of them may seem rather disingenuous of them. People from Western cultures have learned the ethic of "being true to oneself." Swann (1990) has emphasized that people attempt to enact their view of themselves and avoid incorporating the views that others have of them. He calls this motive "self-verification," which is the opposite of symbolic interactionism. In self-verification the self changes others, whereas in symbolic interactionism others change the self. Swann emphasizes the certainty with which a person believes he or she possesses a trait as one variable determining whether a person incorporates the views of others. So if a person feels uncertain about his or her standing on a trait, he or she is more easily influenced by how others see him or her.

So several different theories of self have been presented. They are self-perception ("I see myself as I behave"), self-enhancement ("I see myself as better than others"), self-presentation ("I present myself to others as they want to see me"), and symbolic interactionism ("I see myself as significant others see me") versus self-verification ("I make others see me as I see myself").

Most likely, each of these views of self has some degree of validity. It is incorrect to think that one of them is right and the others are wrong. Moreover, the theories differ in what they concern. Some of the theories concern how knowledge about the self is obtained (e.g., self-perception, symbolic interactionism, and self-verification), whereas other theories are concerned with motives in the evaluation of information (self-enhancement and self-presentation). The knowledge highlighted by these different theoretical perspectives aids us in better understanding the results discussed in this chapter.

Mean Level of Self- versus Other-Perception: Self-Enhancement

What is the difference between self-perception and other-perception? Do people see themselves as better or worse than others? Table 9.2 presents the mean differences between self- and other-perception from four zero-acquaintance studies. Recall that in zero acquaintance the perceiver and target have never interacted. When the numbers in Table 9.2 are positive, people are seeing themselves as better than others; that is, they are self-enhancing. When the numbers are negative, people are seeing others more favorably than themselves.

Most of the numbers in Table 9.2 are positive: People see themselves more favorably than they see others. Because in all these studies the targets being rated are the very same people for both self- and other-ratings, there should be, in principle, no difference between self- and other-ratings. Thus, Table 9.2 presents striking evidence for self-enhancement.

Interestingly, for four of the Big Five factors there is always self-enhancement: People see themselves more favorably than they see others. But for Emotional Stability there is actually self-abasement: People see themselves as more emotionally unstable than they see others. A typical measure of Emotional Stability in these studies is "tense–relaxed" and "anxious–calm." The failure to find self enhancement in ratings of emotional stability provides important evidence against Bem's (1967) self-perception theory. Recall that Bem argued that self- and other-perception both rely on behavioral observation. In these four studies, people probably looked at internal cues and decided that they were anxious and tense. After all, the situation in which they found themselves would be likely to produce anxiety. Recall that

TABLE 9.2. Self-Perception Minus Other-Perception at Zero Acquaintance

Factor	A	B	C	D	Mean
			Study		
Extroversion	.23	.90	.40	.45	.50
Agreeableness	.21	.43	.17	.31	.28
Conscientiousness	.17	.62	.21	.37	.34
Emotional Stability	− .63	− .05	− .62	− .66	− .49
Culture	.09	.62	.17	.41	.32

Note. A, Kenny, Horner, Kashy, and Chu (1992), Study 3; B, Kenny et al. (1992), Study 2; C, Albright, Kenny, and Malloy (1988), Study 3; D, Kenny (1992). Entries reflect differences on a 7-point scale. Positive entries indicate self-enhancement; negative entries indicate self-abasement.

subjects were being rated while they were rating others. But when these people looked at others, those others *appeared* relaxed and calm.

Thus, the results of the zero-acquaintance studies clearly show that people generally engage in self-enhancement: They view themselves more favorably than they view others. But, at least for Emotional Stability, they do also rely on internal cues to which others do not have access.

A key question is whether at higher levels of acquaintance beyond zero acquaintance there is still evidence of self-enhancement. Table 9.3 presents results from three studies in which the perceivers and targets had known each other for a relatively long time. One study was residential (Malloy & Albright, 1990); in this study, the people had known each other for years. In the other two studies, students had been in the same group for a semester.

Averaging across the three studies, one sees self-enhancement on four of the Big Five factors and self-abasement on Emotional Stability. However, the amount of self-enhancement and self-abasement is weaker (i.e., closer to 0) for all five factors. Interestingly, the factor that showed the greatest self-enhancement at zero acquaintance, Extroversion, shows much weaker self-enhancement for well-acquainted individuals. Perhaps because Extroversion is more behavioral than the other factors, it becomes increasingly difficult to self-enhance on that factor. The results from these studies indicate that acquaintance does dilute the self-enhancement and self-abasement effects found at zero acquaintance.

It seems reasonable that there would be less self-enhancement when judging others with whom one has a close relationship. If closeness means incorporating the other as part of the self (Aron & Aron, 1986), then self-ratings should be as positive for ratings of the close other.

TABLE 9.3. Self-Perception Minus Other-Perception among Well-Acquainted Individuals

Factor	Study A	B	C	Mean
Extroversion	.04	.18	.47	.23
Agreeableness	.29	.15	.33	.26
Conscientiousness	.37	.25	.21	.28
Emotional Stability	.31	− .39	− .03	− .04
Culture	.29	.29	.28	.29

Note. A, Malloy and Albright (1990); B, Kenny et al. (1992), Study 3; C, Albright et al. (1988), Study 1. For meaning of entries, see footnote to Table 9.2.

A colleague and I (Kenny & Kashy, in press), for example, found that for some traits, friends were viewed even more positively than self. Thus, in certain cases, perceivers may idealize the targets they are rating.

The results that have been interpreted as indicating self-enhancement might alternatively be viewed as self-presentation effects. That is, people do not actually think that they are better than others; rather, they present themselves to the experimenter as better than others. Although self-presentation is consistent with some results, it cannot easily explain the self-abasement effects found for Emotional Stability. (However, self-handicapping [Berglas & Jones, 1978] explains self-abasement effects within a self-presentation framework.) It then seems likely that the effects that have been discussed are largely attributable to self-enhancement (people think that they are better than others) and not to self-presentation (people want to appear as better than others).

Assumed Similarity

Historically, assumed similarity (Cronbach, 1955) is one of the oldest questions in the field of person perception: Do people see others the way they see themselves? There has been renewed interest in this topic, in that social psychologists have been studying assumed similarity—not only of personality, but also of opinions and behavior. Ross, Greene, and House (1977) have proposed that there is a "false-consensus bias"; that is, people assume that others think, feel, and behave as they do. This book uses the older term of "assumed similarity."

Naively, it seems reasonable that people should see others as they see themselves. So the expectation is for a positive correlation between self-perception and the perceiver effect. However, as reviewed in Chapter 3, there is also a basis for expecting a negative self–perceiver correlation: If people use themselves as a standard in judging others, the more positively they view themselves, the more negatively they should view others.

The easy answer to the question of whether there is assumed similarity is yes. When the perceiver effect is correlated with self-rating, it is virtually always positive. Table 9.4 presents the perceiver–self correlation from four different studies, each of which used the Big Five factors. As the table shows, people tend to see others as they see themselves. Chapter 10 reconsiders the meaning of self–perceiver correlations.

As seen in Table 9.4, the self–perceiver correlations are about .40. The correlations for Extroversion are somewhat lower. Interestingly, the correlations are consistently larger for Agreeableness, averaging about .65. Why are these correlations for Agreeableness so large?

TABLE 9.4. Assumed Similarity: Self–Perceiver Correlations

Factor	Study				
	A	B	C	D	Mean
Extroversion	.23	.42	##	.44	.27
Agreeableness	.62	.82	.43	.74	.65
Conscientiousness	.19	.47	.31	.49	.37
Emotional Stability	.35	.63	.32	.19	.37
Culture	.32	.34	.18	.61	.36

Note. ## = insufficient variance to compute correlation. A, Malloy and Albright (1990); B, Albright et al. (1988), Study 1; C, Malloy (1987a); D, Kenny et al. (1992), Study 2.

One explanation for the assumed similarity for Agreeableness is the reciprocity of prosocial and antisocial behavior, presented in Chapter 6. People who are agreeable probably bring about agreeable behavior in their partners. So if people who see themselves as agreeable are actually agreeable, their interaction partners should also be agreeable. So it is reasonable for agreeable people to expect others to be agreeable. Although this reciprocity hypothesis is plausible, there is no direct test of it.

An alternate and simpler explanation is assumed reciprocity.[1] If a person believes that he or she is agreeable, the person may assume that others are also agreeable when they are with him or her. Alternatively, the person may see himself or herself as not so agreeable because he or she assumes that others are hostile. (See the discussions of complementary projection in Chapters 3, 6, and 10.) Evidently, reciprocity is not assumed as much for the other Big Five factors.

As discussed in Chapter 3, the perceiver effect is likely to be contaminated by response set. No doubt the overwhelming evidence for assumed similarity partially reflects the presence of the same response set in self- and other-ratings. The question of assumed similarity and its relation to response set is discussed in the final chapter of the book.

Relative Amount of Perceiver Variance in Self- and Other-Ratings

Recall that in Chapter 3, the perceiver effect has been conceptualized as a measure of ignorance. It represents a person's best guess of what people are like. It seems sensible that the perceiver effect should be weighted less in self-perception, in that people presumably know themselves well.

A method is needed to evaluate how the self and others weight the perceiver effect. In other-perception, how Zelda sees Heidi is assumed to be a function of Zelda's perceiver effect and of Heidi's target effect. Self-perception too can be assumed to be a function of perceiver and target effects, but those effects may not be weighted as they are in other-perception.

Consider the Social Relations Model (SRM) equation for perceiver i rating target j:

$$X_{ij} = m + a_i + b_j + g_{ij}$$

As explained in Chapter 2 and Appendix B, m is the constant, a_i is the perceiver effect, b_j is person j's target effect, and g_{ij} is the relationship effect. The model for person i's self-rating (i's rating of i, or X_{ii}) is as follows:

$$X_{ii} = n + ka_i + qb_i + h_{ii}$$

This equation for self-perception looks very much like the traditional SRM specification, but there are some important differences. First, note that the perceiver and target are the very same person, and so i and j are the same; hence X_{ii}. Second, the constant and relationship effects are different from what they are in the equation for other-perception. Third, both the perceiver and the target effects that are present in other-perception are also present in self-perception; however, these effects may be weighted differently for self-perception. The parameter that multiplies the perceiver effect is k, and the parameter that multiplies the target effect is q. The parameter k is the assumed-similarity parameter, and the parameter q is the one for self–other agreement, which is discussed later in this chapter.

In essence, the parameter k states the relative amount of perceiver variance in self-perception versus other-perception. Consider the case in which there are self- and other-perceptions of friendliness. If k is bigger than 1, then the perceiver effect has more weight in self-perception than in other-perception. So if a person tends to see others as friendly, the person should see himself or herself as even more friendly. If k is less than 1, then the perceiver effect has less weight in self-perception than in other-perception. So if a person sees others as friendly, the person should see himself or herself as not quite that friendly. If k is 1, then the perceiver effect is weighted in self-perception as it is in other-perception. If k is zero, then the perceiver effect is not used at all in self-perception. So how a person sees others has no relationship to how the person sees himself or herself. Finally, if k is negative,

TABLE 9.5. The Relative Weight (k) of the Perceiver Effect in Self-Perception

| | Study | | | | |
Factor	A	B	C	D	Median
Extroversion	1.10	.61	##	##	.86
Agreeableness	.70	.74	1.17	.99	.84
Conscientiousness	.60	.70	.95	—	.70
Emotional Stability	.56	.70	.71	—	.70
Culture	1.75	.64	.78	.78	.78

Note. ## = insufficient variance to compute weight. — = factor not measured. A, Malloy and Albright (1990); B, Albright et al. (1988), Study 1; C, Malloy (1987a); D, Levesque (1990).

then others are seen as different from the self. So if a person sees others as friendly, the person sees himself or herself as unfriendly.

Now that a measure of the weight of the perceiver effect in self-perception has been developed, what is that weight? Table 9.5 presents the value of k from four studies. As seen in the table, k tends to be greater than zero and less than 1. The typical value of k is about .75. So perceivers are using the perceiver effect in self-perception, but it has less influence in self-perception than it does in other-perception. If the perceiver effect is viewed as a general stereotype of others (see Chapter 3), people do not believe that the stereotype applies as much to them as it does to others.

Acquaintance and Assumed Similarity

Chapter 3 has also discussed the perceiver effect as the perceiver's stereotype of the group being rated. It seems reasonable to believe that as a person remains in a group for a longer time, the person should come to see group members as he or she sees himself or herself. Research on ingroup versus outgroup perceptions has shown that people often assume that ingroup members (their own group) are more similar to them than are outgroup members (the other group).

Table 9.6 presents the self–perceiver correlation at varying levels of acquaintance. The table very convincingly shows that increasing acquaintance leads to greater assumed similarity. For all three studies presented, the self–perceiver correlation increases with increasing acquaintance. Interestingly, the self–perceiver correlations are smallest for the Park and Judd (1989) study, which had the least amount of interaction between subjects.

In a cross-sectional study, we (Kenny & Kashy, in press) com-

TABLE 9.6. Assumed Similarity (Self–Perceiver Correlation) and Mean Liking for Increasing Acquaintance

Study	Assumed similarity	Mean liking
Montgomery (1984) (2 traits)		
Wave 1	.51	5.01
Wave 2	.70	5.24
Wave 3	.72	5.18
Albright-Malloy (1988) (5 traits)		
Wave 1	.59	5.60
Wave 2	.58	5.90
Wave 3	.81	5.80
Park & Judd (1989) (14 traits)		
Wave 1	.15	4.95
Wave 2	.30	4.78
Wave 3	.29	4.80
Wave 4	.36	4.88

puted the self–perceiver correlation in ratings of friends and acquaintances. For all four traits that we examined, the self–perceiver correlation was greater for ratings of friends than of acquaintances. This result too is consistent with the view that acquaintance leads to greater self–perceiver correlations.

So as a person gets to know someone better and presumably likes that other more, the person sees the other as more similar to himself or herself. Table 9.6 also presents the mean liking at each time point. Liking does somewhat increase with increasing acquaintance, and so there is limited support for the hypothesis that a presumed moderator of assumed similarity is liking. However, because the liking means do not exactly parallel the assumed-similarity correlations, it may be true that another factor besides liking explains the increase in assumed similarity with increasing acquaintance. Perhaps familiarity itself leads to assumed similarity.

Self–Other Agreement

There are two individual-difference terms in SRM: perceiver and target. The preceding section has considered the overlap in self-perception and the perceiver effect. This section considers the overlap between the target effect and self-perception.

The question of self–other agreement is a fundamental question in social science. As discussed in Chapter 7, self-ratings are often used as criterion measures in accuracy research, and so the self–other correlation is often taken as a measure of accuracy. Also, symbolic interactionists have claimed that people come to see themselves as other people do. Self-other correlations (Shrauger & Schoeneman, 1979) have played an important role in testing symbolic interactionism.

Level of Self–Other Agreement

Before self–other agreement can be measured, it first needs to be established that peers do agree with each other. If peers do not agree, how can it be expected that the self would agree with peers? So consensus or agreement between peers, the topic of Chapter 4, is a necessary condition for self–other agreement. In the tables in this section of the chapter, self–other agreement is not computed unless at least 10% of the variance in other-perceptions is at the level of the target. If this criterion is not reached, the symbol "##" is used, indicating that there is not enough meaningful variation in the target effect for the self–other correlation to be computed.

In an influential review of the literature, Shrauger and Schoeneman (1979) surveyed many studies that measured the level of the self–other correlation. They concluded that "there is no persistent agreement between people's self-perceptions and how they are actually viewed by others" (p. 549). However, their often-cited conclusion is misleading. If one examines their own data, the average self–other correlation (using the Fisher's z transformation) across 31 studies is not zero, but equals about .27. Shrauger and Schoeneman (1979) judged this correlation as small because they compared it to the correlation between how people see themselves and how they think others see them. As reviewed in Chapter 8 (see especially Table 8.7), this latter correlation is very large and often approaches 1 when corrections for unreliability are made. Thus, Shrauger and Schoeneman (1979) placed an unfair burden on the self–other correlation; their own data actually support a moderate self-other correlation.

Work by Funder (1980), Funder and Colvin (1988), McCrae and Costa (1989), John and Robins (1993), and Kenrick and Funder (1988) has consistently found a correlation between how people see themselves and how others see them. However, none of these studies employed an SRM analysis, and so their results must be interpreted with some degree of caution (Kenny & Albright, 1987).

Table 9.7 presents self–other correlations from four different

TABLE 9.7. Self–Other Agreement (Self–Target Correlation) among Highly Acquainted Persons

	Big Five factor				
	I	II	III	IV	V
Kenny et al. (1992), Study 3	.66	.49	1.00	##	##
Malloy & Albright (1990)	.48	.36	.38	.52	.38
Dantchik (1985)	.78	.71	.40	.12	.62
Albright (1990)	.74	.12	.09	.44	.51
Median	.70	.42	.39	.44	.51

Note. ## – insufficient variance to compute correlation. Factor numbers in this and subsequent tables: I, Extroversion; II, Agreeableness; III, Conscientiousness; IV, Emotional Stability; V, Culture.

studies in which the judges and targets had known each other for an extended time. (Correlations for other levels of acquaintance are considered later in this chapter.) In three of the four studies, the judges and the targets lived in the same residential unit; in one study, the research participants were members of a class and had known one another for a semester. The data in all four studies were analyzed using SRM, and for each study the correlations are computed for each of the Big Five factors.

Table 9.7 very convincingly shows that for Extroversion (Factor I), others do indeed see people as they see themselves. The "smallest" correlation is .48, and the median is .70. For Extroversion, there is close but not perfect correspondence between self-perception and other-perception. For the other four factors, there is not much consistency; some studies show large correlations and others do not. Across all the studies, the median correlation is .42 for all the factors but Extroversion. This value is somewhat larger than the .27 value from the 31 studies reviewed by Shrauger and Schoeneman (1979). But because the correlations in Table 9.7 have been corrected for unreliability (i.e., they are a forecast of what the correlation would be if an infinite number of perceivers were to evaluate the target), whereas the Shrauger and Schoeneman correlations were not, the expectation is for the Shrauger and Schoeneman correlations to be somewhat smaller than the correlations in Table 9.7. So except for Extroversion, the results in Table 9.7 are pretty much in line with the results (if not the conclusion) of Shrauger and Schoeneman (1979). Thus, self–other agreement is about .7 for Extroversion and about .4 for the other four factors. In summary, both the data presented by Shrauger and Schoeneman (1979) and the results from four SRM analyses strongly support the conclusion that people do indeed see themselves as others do.

Consensus versus Self–Other Agreement

Even if it is known that the self agrees with peers, it can be asked whether peers agree more with each other than the self agrees with peers. So, for example, do Curly and Larry agree more in their ratings of Moe than Moe's self-rating agrees with the rating of Curly or Larry?

Measurement Issues

The simplest way to answer this question is to compare two correlations: the self–peer and the peer–peer correlations. A better way to make this comparison is to use the weight q, discussed earlier in this chapter. If self-ratings correlate more highly with other-ratings than other-ratings do with each other, then q should be greater than 1. However, if self-ratings correlate less with other-ratings than other-atings correlate with each other, then the weight q should be less than 1. If the coefficient is 1, then peer–peer agreement is as great as self–peer agreement. If the coefficient is greater than one, then perhaps the self has some special insight that peers can only partially see. Finally, if the coefficient is negative, people see the person very differently from the way the person sees himself or herself.

Empirical Review

Table 9.8 presents the value of q for five studies that examined ratings of physical attractiveness. This variable is chosen because it shows reasonable levels of consensus, even when the perceiver and target are not well acquainted. As the table clearly shows, because the values of q are generally less than 1, self-ratings agree less with other-ratings than do other-ratings agree with each other. So at least for physical attractiveness, the evidence is that peers agree more with each other than they do with the self.

Theoretical Explanation

There are at least three possible explanations of why peers agree more with each other than they do with the self. First, self-ratings may be so positively inflated that there is a ceiling effect: People actually have, or they present to others, a very inflated image of themselves. Thus, self-ratings cannot correlate very highly with the ratings that others give. At least for ratings of physical attractiveness, however, this ceiling effect explanation is not plausible. The mean rating of physical

TABLE 9.8. Relative Weight of Self–Peer Agreement versus
Peer–Peer Agreement for Perceptions of Physical Attractiveness

Study	Weight
Albright et al. (1988), Study 3	.43
Latané (1987)	.50
Kenny et al. (1992), Study 2	.37
Kenny et al. (1992), Study 3	
Wave 0	.34
Wave 1	− .05
Park & Judd (1989)	
Wave 1	.96
Wave 2	.67
Wave 3	.55
Wave 4	.64

Note. A weight less than 1 implies greater peer–peer agreement than self–peer agreement.

attractiveness is not very different from the average rating given to others. It is true that in all but one study presented in Table 9.8, the self-rating mean is greater than the mean rating of others, but the difference between the two ratings is generally rather small. Never does the self-rating of attractiveness approach the ceiling or upper limit.

The second explanation of greater agreement between peers than that between a peer and the self is that peers communicate with each other, and that is why they agree more. This explanation is not viable for most of the studies in Table 9.8, because the peers never interacted with one another and so had no opportunity to communicate. It should be realized that communication can also potentially bias the self–peer correlation: Peers may influence the self and the self may influence peers (see the section below on self-verification).

The third explanation is that peers use different cues than the self uses. Peers have limited information that they use in making judgments, but that limited information is generally publicly observable. The self has other information that he or she can evaluate; in particular, the self can examine internal states and the past to make judgments. Most likely, the fundamental reason why peers agree more with each other than with the self is that, in making self-judgments, people's self-theories are less grounded in currently observable reality than are peer judgments. The often-made statement that attractive fashion models frequently have negative self-images is consistent with the results in Table 9.8.

If self-ratings are based less on observable behavior than other-ratings are, then it is quite ironic that self-ratings are often used as the standard to judge other-ratings, in that other-ratings may be more valid than self-ratings. The question of the relative validity of self- versus other-ratings is considered in a later section.

The reader might wonder whether the results in Table 9.8 are unique to judgments of physical attractiveness. Generally for other traits besides physical attractiveness, the weights are usually less than 1, which indicates that peers agree more with each other than they do with the self. As an example, Table 9.9 presents results for the Big Five factors from four studies. As seen in the table, the weights tend to be less than 1, so the results for attractiveness in Table 9.8 are not aberrant. There does appear to be an exception, though: For Factor V, Culture, the coefficients tend to be larger than 1. Although clearly more research is needed, the self may have more insight than others do into this factor.

Weighted-Average Model of Perception

Because the present topic is how self-perception differs from other-perception, it should be possible to specify within the Weighted-Average Model (WAM), developed in Chapter 4, the exact nature of these differences.[2] Using this model reveals that there are four potential differences between self- and other-perception.

First, the self has observed many thousands (perhaps millions!) of the self's own acts, whereas others cannot have observed so many acts. This fact suggests that the self should, in principle, agree with peers less than peers agree with each other if there is some overlap in the acts observed by peers (and if the consistency parameter is not too large).

Second, because the self has seen so many acts, self-perception should be less influenced by physical appearance than other-perception

TABLE 9.9. Relative Weight of Self–Peer Agreement versus Peer–Peer Agreement for Ratings of the Big Five Factors

	Big Five factor				
Study	I	II	III	IV	V
Malloy & Albright (1990)	.84	.02	.57	.70	1.82
Dantchik (1985)	1.85	1.01	.98	.33	1.19
Levesque (1990)	.76	.28	—	—	1.16
Kenny et al. (1992), Study 3	.50	– .82	.35	– .79	##

Note. — = factor not measured. ## = insufficient variance to measure weight. A weight less than 1 implies greater peer–peer agreement than self–peer agreement.

should be. Peer ratings are more influenced by physical appearance, and presumably there is close agreement in the evaluation of the physical-appearance information.

Third, self-perception may be dramatically influenced by communication effects from parents and other significant people. Because these people are not likely to influence the peers' ratings of the person, this too should lead to lowered self–peer agreement.

Finally, the unique impression may have a very large influence in self-perception. That is, the self-evaluation may be determined not only by behavior and appearance, but also by an emotional evaluation of the self. Peer perception may be more "objective," in that the unique impression has much less weight than it does for self-perception.

Summary

In summary, it seems that peers agree more with each other than they do with the self. The likely reason for this result is that peer ratings are more closely tied to the target's current behavior, whereas self-ratings are more closely tied to deep-seated self-theories that may not have limited current behavioral validity. The next section considers the question of the relative validity of peer perceptions versus self-perceptions. The expectation, based on the results of these analyses, is that peer ratings should be more valid than self-ratings.

Relative Validity of Peer and Self-Ratings

Besides the level of self–other correlation, a related question can be asked: Whose reports are more valid, the self's or peers'? If a person's friend thinks that the person is lazy, but the person himself or herself does not, who is right? Before the evidence is examined, an important methodological point should be made. In comparing the relative validity of self and peer, the researcher should be careful not to use peer reports that are averaged across multiple peers. If aggregated peer reports are used, they would probably appear to be more valid than self-reports only because they are more reliable. If peer reports are aggregated measures, appropriate psychometric corrections must be made to take into account data aggregation.

Would we expect peers or the self to be more valid? The naive answer is that the self should be more valid, because the self has access to much more information than do peers. In particular, the self has access to internal states to which others do not have easy access. On the other hand, self-perception is subject to a host of biases, most notably self-enhancement. So we might think that self-ratings are less valid than are ratings of a knowledgeable informant.

Unfortunately, there is not much evidence concerning the relative validity of peer perception versus self-perception. What little work there is points to greater validity in other-ratings than in self-ratings, but these studies do have limitations. Three different studies can shed some light on the relative validity of self- versus other-ratings. In one of these studies (Levesque & Kenny, 1993; described in detail in Chapter 7), subjects predicted the behavior of their future interaction partners, with whom they then interacted one-on-one. In the other studies (John & Robins, 1994, and Shechtman, 1994), subjects postdicted the behavior of their partners with whom they had interacted in a group. In all but the Levesque and Kenny (1993) study, the self-ratings were ratings of how the person behaved in the interactions. That is, the person was instructed to rate how he or she behaved in the particular interaction, instead of how he or she is in general.

For all three studies, the correlation between other-perceptions and ratings by trained observers was greater than the correlation between self-ratings and observer ratings. Thus, these studies showed that others were better able to predict behavior than the self. What is even more remarkable is that the perceivers in these studies were initially strangers.

There are two major limitations in these studies. First, the criterion was the behavior that the peers directly observed. The self evidently used past behaviors in perceiving the current behaviors, and peers did not. Self-ratings might be more valid if the criterion were to predict behavior in a different setting. Second, in these studies the observers were, in a sense, peers. So it is not very surprising that two types of peers agreed more than the self and a peer did (see above analysis). Following the analysis of Kruglanski (1989), it can be asked why an observer should be the standard setter and not the self.

Although more research is needed, the best current evidence is that other-ratings are as valid as, if not more valid than, self-ratings if the criterion is the observation of trained observers. This result should lead researchers to question seriously the orientation that views personality as the study of self-report inventories. These inventories are predictive of self-views, but may be less useful in predicting behavior. Certainly for some variables, the self should be more accurate than others; for instance, the self is probably more accurate at reporting emotional states and attitudes than are others. But for perceptions of personality, knowledgeable others may be more valid than the self.

Moderators of Self–Other Agreement

What factors lead to greater self–other agreement? This section considers observability, evaluative extremity, and acquaintance as possible moderators of self–other agreement.

Observability

In their important paper, Kenrick and Stringfield (1980) claimed that a significant moderator of self–other agreement is "observability." The more observable the trait, the more likely it is that the self and peers will agree. Others have pursued the Kenrick and Stringfield hypothesis,[3] but they have used other terms besides "observable": "external," "behavioral," "confirmable," "specific," and so on. Funder and Dobroth (1987) have empirically shown that there is considerable overlap in the meanings of these terms.

One reason why observability appears to be a moderator of the self–other correlation is that self–other agreement is much higher for Extroversion than it is for other traits. If Extroversion traits were removed from the list, perhaps observability would not be as closely related to self–other agreement. In the model of consensus presented in Chapter 4, observability comes closest to the parameter called "similar meaning systems" or r_2. Presumably, to the extent to which the trait being rated is less closely tied to behavior (i.e., is less observable), there should be less consensus and also less self–other agreement.

Evaluative Extremity

In perhaps the most extensive search for moderators of the self–other correlation, John and Robins (1993) examined a whole host of possible moderators. They found that evaluative extremity is the strongest moderator of the difference between the self–other and the peer–peer correlations. Traits that are evaluatively extreme are those traits for which people will very much like or dislike targets possessing that trait. For instance, "honest–dishonest" is high on evaluative extremity, whereas "organized–disorganized" is not. Most people will like an honest person and dislike a dishonest person, but most people will neither like nor dislike an organized person.

John and Robins (1993) reasoned that people who are judged by others as scoring high on evaluatively extreme traits ("saints") should rate themselves modestly, whereas people who are negatively judged by others ("jerks") should try to present themselves favorably. So

evaluatively extreme traits should have relatively low self–other agreement, because saints should underestimate their true standing and jerks
should overestimate it. For traits that are not evaluatively extreme, there
should be no such bias. John and Robins present strong evidence that
evaluative extremity moderates self–other agreement. The self, then,
may not provide very valid ratings when traits are evaluatively extreme.
It should be realized that most personality traits are evaluatively extreme (Borkenau, 1990); that is, neutral traits are relatively rare.

Earlier, in Table 9.7, it has been shown that Extroversion shows
the greatest self–other agreement. This would appear to be consistent
with the work of John and Robins (1993) in that Extroversion is less
evaluatively extreme than the other factors.

Acquaintance

Does self–other agreement change as a function of acquaintance? Correlations from a paper by McCrae (1982) are often cited as showing high
self–other agreement in people who are well acquainted with each other
(spouses). Their nondisattenuated self–other correlations average about
.59, which is larger than the typical self–other correlation (see Table
9.7). However, as discussed in both Chapters 4 and 7, those correlations are probably inflated. Because spouses are similar to each other
on a whole host of characteristics, and because people often assume
similarity (e.g., see Table 9.4), the combination of actual and assumed
similarity creates, in part, the high self–other agreement found in married couples. By using multiple-partner designs, researchers can
eliminate the assumed-similarity explanation of self–other agreement.

Table 9.10 presents the self–other correlation at zero acquaintance and is adapted from Albright, Malloy, Kenny, and Borkenau
(1994). Again, note that many entries in the table are given as "##,"
which means that there is insufficient target variance or consensus to
compute the self–other correlation. The table impressively demonstrates
that, at least for Extroversion and Conscientiousness, there is a
self–other correlation even at zero acquaintance. For the other three
factors, there is no evidence of a correlation between self- and other-
perception, because there is not sufficient target variance for a correlation to be computed.

The self–other correlations at zero acquaintance point to evidence
for a "kernel of truth" effect. Evidently the stereotypes held at zero
acquaintance have some degree of validity. The Levesque and Kenny
(1993) study presented in Chapter 7 provides further evidence of the
kernel of truth for Extroversion judgments.

A comparison of the results from Table 9.7 and Table 9.10 indi-

TABLE 9.10. Self–Other Agreement (Self–Target Correlation) at Zero Acquaintance

Study	Big Five factor				
	I	II	III	IV	V
Albright et al. (1988), Study 1	.44	##	.52	.01	−.19
Albright et al. (1988), Study 2	.33	##	.52	##	##
Albright et al. (1988), Study 3	.34	##	.34	##	##
Borkenau and Liebler (1992)	.41	.06	.33	.02	.05
DiPilato (1990)	.49	##	##	.00	##
Kenny (1992)	.49	##	##	##	##
Kenny et al. (1992), Study 1	.03	.09	.20	##	##
Kenny et al. (1992), Study 2	.33	##	.02	##	##
Kenny et al. (1992), Study 3	.62	##	##	##	##
Latané (1987)	—	.16	.58	—	−.28

Note. ## = less than 10% of the variance attributable to target. — = factor not measured. Adapted from Albright, Kenny, Malloy, and Borkenau (1994). Used by permission of the authors.

cates that at zero acquaintance, the self–target correlation for Extroversion averages .35, whereas for well-acquainted people the average correlation rises to .66. So at least for Extroversion, there is a relationship between acquaintance and self–other agreement. There is only a trivial increase for Conscientiousness: The correlation averages about .36 at zero acquaintance and only rises to .39 for those well acquainted.

Three longitudinal studies have shown an increase in the self–other correlation as a function of acquaintance (Park & Judd, 1989; Paulhus & Bruce, 1992; Montgomery, 1984). All three of these were group studies; that is, the subjects interacted in groups and not one-on-one. Interestingly, the Paulhus and Bruce (1992) study shows a decline in consensus over time with increasing self–other agreement. The self–target correlations from Park and Judd (1989) generally increase across the 4 days of the study: .09, .28, .42, and .38. This pattern of results is further evidence that increased acquaintance does lead to increased self–other agreement. Surprisingly, the only study of people living together (Albright, 1990) has not shown increasing self–other correlations. It may be that self–other agreement peaks relatively quickly during the acquaintance process.

Further support for the hypothesis that increases in acquaintance lead to greater self–other agreement is provided by a recent study (Kenny & Kashy, in press). We found that self-ratings correlated more strongly with a friend's rating of the person than with an acquaintance's. The evidence supports the proposition that increasing acquaintance leads to greater self–other agreement. However, the absence of a longitudinal, residential study supporting this hypothesis is somewhat disquieting.

Theories of Self–Other Agreement

It is standard practice to teach beginning students in the social and behavioral sciences the following dictum: "Correlation does not imply causality." If it is found that two variables, say X and Y, are correlated, this does not imply that X causes Y. There are three alternate causal explanations of any correlation:

1. X causes Y.
2. Y causes X.
3. Z causes both X and Y.

Each of these three different explanations can account for self–other agreement. So it is possible that (1) other-perception causes self-perception; (2) self-perception causes other-perception; or (3) both are caused by another variable. These three explanations of the self–other correlation are now considered.

Other-Perception Causes Self-Perception

First, how others see a person may influence that person to see himself or herself in the same way. The hypothesis that we see ourselves as others see us has been put forth by symbolic interactionists. (Symbolic interactionism has been previously discussed in Chapter 8 and earlier in this chapter.) These theorists, drawing on the pioneering work of Mead and Cooley, argue that the self is created from how others see the person; actually, it is not just any others, but significant others that matter. These significant others are defined by the person, but generally they include parents and close friends.

As previously reviewed in Chapter 8, evidence for the symbolic-interactionist view of self-perception is rather thin. The sociologist Richard Felson has shown that significant others do not have as much of an effect as might be thought. In one study, Felson (1981) showed that high school football players' evaluations of their performance did not resemble their coaches' evaluations of their performance. Symbolic interactionists may argue that Felson did not study "significant" others; however, Felson carefully argued that coaches are indeed significant others.

An alternate view is that the self-concept may be fixed early in life and is difficult to change in adulthood. In a longitudinal study,

Felson (1989) found evidence that parents do affect a child's self-concept.

Self-Perception Causes Other-Perception

Second, how a person views himself or herself may influence others to see him or her that way. As noted earlier, Swann (1990) has argued that individuals engage in a process called "self-verification." People have a strong motive to seek to have others see them as they see themselves. Part of the self-verification motive is an attempt, either conscious or unconscious, to persuade others to see one as one sees oneself. People are very invested in their self-images, and they want others to bolster those self-images. Swann (1990) has amassed an impressive body of evidence that people seek out confirmation of their self-images. Surprisingly, self-verification occurs even when an individual's self-image is negative. Identity is a precarious quality that needs support, even if the self-perceptions are what most people would consider destructive.

How does a person communicate his or her self-concept to others? First, there is communication by physical appearance; people use clothes, jewelry, and hair styles to express their self-images. Second, people directly communicate aspects of themselves to others through self-disclosure. Self-disclosure, thought to be important in relationship development, also serves the function of self-verification.

As Swann (1990) sees it, it is more important to verify one's identity to some targets than to others. Close others reinforce the image of self better than complete strangers do. When a person's self-concept is threatened, the person often seeks out intimates to bolster his or her self-image (Swann & Predmore, 1985). Indeed, people may seek out as friends those who confirm their identities, and discard others who view them differently from the way they view themselves. If this is true, then self–other agreement should be stronger for friends than for ordinary others —a result consistent with our findings (Kenny & Kashy, in press).

People seek to verify aspects of themselves that they are confident are true. But if people are not confident about certain aspects of themselves, they need others to tell them their standing on these traits. So Swann (1990) believes that confidence provides a reconciliation between the influence of others and self-verification. Self-verification operates when the self is certain, and symbolic interactionism operates when the self is uncertain.

Both Are Caused by Another Variable

Third, it may well be that some other factor or factors determine both self- and other-perception. According to Bem's (1967) self-perception theory as described earlier, self-perception is little different from other-perception; in both cases, people observe their own behavior and make inferences. Within social psychology, Felson (1980, 1981), the critic of symbolic interactionism, has been the major proponent of the hypothesis that self- and other-perception have a common cause. Some of this research has been reviewed in Chapter 8.

Consider a simple example. How do college students know how smart they are? They take courses, are tested, and receive grades. They use this information to form a view of themselves. Others also use this information to form a judgment of the students' intelligence. So grades and test performance—external cues—largely determine both self- and other-perceptions of the intelligence of college students.

The self and others do not always use valid information in making judgments; they may also use invalid sources. Both self- and other-perceptions are also influenced by social stereotypes. Racial, sexual, ethnic, and age stereotypes no doubt play an important role in other-perception. These stereotypes also presumably affect self-perceptions. So the correlation between the perceptions of self and others reflects, in part, the shared use of social stereotypes in personality judgments.

So, the self and other can agree, yet neither may be influencing the other. It is obvious that self and other agree that the sky is blue, but in this instance few would think that agreement is due to influence. Self and other can agree because they are perceiving the same reality.

Summary of Theories

Causation between self- and other-perception certainly may run in all possible directions. At least for adults, causation does not typically flow from others to the self. Self-verification has been shown to operate, at least when the self feels certain about his or her views. However, it seems most plausible that the major reason for self–other agreement is that both self and other are using the self's behavior to form judgments.

Variability in Self- versus Other-Ratings

Jones and Nisbett (1971) defined the "actor–observer effect" as follows: People see other people's behavior as dispositionally caused and their own behavior as situationally determined. One implication of the actor–observer effect is that there should be more variability in other-ratings than in self-ratings. If people see themselves as situationally determined, they should not see themselves as very extreme on traits. However, if people see others' behavior as dispositionally caused, they should see others as extreme. Because extremity is closely tied to variability, the actor–observer effect implies more variance in other-perception than in self-perception.

Earlier in this chapter, the relationship effect for self-ratings has been defined as the self-rating minus the perceiver and target effects, each weighted appropriately. (Recall that the weight for the perceiver effect is denoted as k and the weight for the target effect as q.) This relationship effect in self-perception measures how the person sees himself or herself differently from how he or she sees others and differently from how others see him or her.

Table 9.11 presents the results from several studies of the relative amounts of relationship variance in self-ratings versus other-ratings. The table merely indicates whether there is more relationship variance in self- or in other-ratings. If there is more variance in self-ratings, there is an "S," and if there is more variance in other-ratings, there is an "O."

For the three zero-acquaintance studies, the pattern is fairly clear: There tends to be more relationship variance in self-ratings than in other-ratings. Beyond zero acquaintance, the pattern is less than clear-cut. The evidence seems to point to basically the same amount of relationship variance in other- and self-ratings. Thus, the results in Table 9.11 provide no support for the actor–observer effect. On the contrary, when the perceivers do not know the targets well, perceivers see more variability in themselves than in others.

Conclusion

Research on the self has a long history in social science. Many theories have been developed to explain self-perception, most notably

TABLE 9.11. Preponderance of Self (S) or Other (O) Relationship Variance

Study	Big Five factor				
	I	II	III	IV	V
Zero acquaintance					
Albright et al. (1988), Study 1	S	S	S	S	O
Kenny et al. (1992), Study 2	O	O	S	S	S
Kenny et al. (1992), Study 3	S	O	S	S	O
Perceiver and target acquainted					
Levesque (1990)	O	O	—	—	O
Kenny et al. (1992), Study 2	S	O	S	S	O
Kenny et al. (1992), Study 3	S	O	S	O	S

Note. — = factor not measured.

self-perception theory, self-enhancement bias, self-presentation theory, symbolic interactionism, and self-verification.

Consistent with the self-enhancement and self-presentation theories, it is found that people see themselves more favorably than others see them. Inconsistent with self-perception theory, self-deprecation is found for Emotional Stability. These self-enhancement and self-abasement effects weaken as people become more acquainted.

Self-ratings carry a great deal of excess baggage; that is, they measure other things besides how the person truly is. Self-ratings may better reflect a person's past behavior (which was probably shaped by parental expectations) than the person's current personality. That is, people may fail to update their self-perceptions with current information. Also, people fail to realize how much their behavior changes from situation to situation and from partner to partner; they think that they are more consistent than they really are.

These false self-perceptions can even be fatal. People with anorexia nervosa may starve themselves to death because they see themselves as the heavier persons they used to be. Successful people may commit suicide because they see themselves as failures in their parents' eyes.

Self-ratings are also considerably distorted by self-presentation, by response set, and by self-enhancement. As suggested in Chapter 7, researchers should stop using self-ratings as criterion scores for target accuracy, and instead should use behavioral ratings.

Self-ratings are not totally invalid, because they agree with the ratings of others. There are three possible sources of this agreement: Other-ratings may cause self-ratings (symbolic interactionism); self-ratings may cause other-ratings (self-verification); and both may be caused by the person's behavior (Bem's self-perception theory). It would appear that the bulk of the agreement is attributable to the fact that both self- and other-ratings are caused by the behavior of the person being rated. However, not enough research has been done to permit a definitive statement on this issue.

The next chapter of this book, the final one, summarizes and ties together themes that cut across the other chapters.

Notes

1. I want to acknowledge Maurice Levesque, who first suggested this idea to me.

2. I want to acknowledge Michiko Nohara, who first suggested this idea to me.

3. Actually, Kenrick and Stringfield (1980) discussed observability as a between-person variable, not as a factor that differentiates traits.

Chapter 10

REVIEW AND INTEGRATION

This chapter attempts to tie together the results that have been presented in the previous chapters. In those chapters, it has often been necessary to separate artificially processes that are necessarily interrelated; in this chapter, the material is integrated. The present chapter also provides the opportunity to reflect on the limits and potential of the Weighted-Average Model (WAM), the Social Relations Model (SRM), and the notational system. Moreover, it provides an opportunity to examine the relationship between perception and behavior.

The chapter is divided into five sections. In the first section, the answers to the nine basic questions are reviewed. The second part of the chapter considers WAM. The third part discusses the limits of SRM. The fourth part reviews the notational system developed in Chapter 1 and presents some possible extensions. The last part of this chapter extensively analyzes the relationship between perception and behavior.

Summary of Results

Assimilation

The perceiver effect reflects the tendency for a person to see targets as similar, or assimilation. Assimilation is symbolized by $Z(H) = Z(C)$. About 20% of the total variance in the perception of others is attributable to the perceiver. The perceiver effect reflects more than how people assign numbers to other people; it seems to reflect how the rater views the particular group that is being judged, and so it represents the person's differential stereotype for the group. This stereotype explanation of the perceiver effect is bolstered by evidence that assimilation declines as the perceiver gets to know the targets better. Also, as the perceiver begins to identify with the group, the perceiver effect reflects how the person sees himself or herself.

Consensus

The target effect reflects the tendency for perceivers to agree, or consensus. Consensus is symbolized by $Z(H) = C(H)$. There is consensus in interpersonal perception, in that perceivers do agree when they evaluate a common target. However, even among highly acquainted people, consensus explains less than a third of the total variance. On average, about 15% of the total variance reflects consensus. Consensus exists even before people interact. There is evidence that Extroversion judgments are more consensual than other judgments, especially when acquaintance is low.

Surprisingly, there is little or no relationship between consensus and acquaintance. One reason for the failure to find longitudinal trends is that initially stereotypes (which are highly consensual) are used to form impressions, and this brings about consensus; later, behavioral information is used, but its meaning is much less consensual. Moreover, in most studies of the relationship between acquaintance and consensus, there is high information overlap; that is, all of the perceivers have access to the same information about the targets. In situations of high overlap, WAM predicts little or no relationship between acquaintance and consensus. For these reasons, with greater acquaintance there is not necessarily an increase in consensus.

Uniqueness

Uniqueness in perception is reflected in the relationship effect. It is symbolized by $Z(H) <> Z(C)$ and $Z(H) <> C(H)$. About 20% of the total variance is attributable to the relationship. Uniqueness seems virtually always to characterize interpersonal perception; a major challenge in future work is to comprehend the meaning of this component. Other-perception is quite idiosyncratic, yet researchers in interpersonal perception have little understanding about why there is uniqueness.

One possible explanation is that the same person takes on different roles with different partners. The same person is a child, a best friend, a teammate, a casual acquaintance, a classmate, an enemy, and a roommate to different people. Perhaps much of the relationship variance reflects the different roles that people take on in social life (Kashy, 1992; Steiner, 1955). Targets are viewed in terms of their role relationships with the perceivers, and the meaning of those relationships is largely culturally based.

Assumed and Actual Reciprocity

Reciprocity in perception is symbolized by $Z(H) = H(Z)$ and assumed reciprocity by $Z(H) = Z(H(Z))$. There is little or no indication of reciprocity, either perceived or actual, in trait perception. There is some indication, however, that Agreeableness is reciprocated at the individual level. That is, people who are seen by others as agreeable see those others as agreeable. This reciprocation in perception is probably caused by an underlying reciprocity of prosocial and antisocial behavior.

Target Accuracy

Target accuracy refers to the degree to which other-perceptions are valid, and is symbolized by $Z(H) = H$. Research on target accuracy is quite difficult because of problems concerning the separation of both the perception and the criterion into components, as well as the measurement of the criterion. Initial research provides evidence for generalized accuracy in the rating of Extroversion. The consensual judgments of Extroversion made at zero acquaintance agree with self-perception and are accurate. We (Levesque & Kenny, 1993) have speculated that the quick consensus on Extroversion may reflect the survival value of identifying leaders in moments of crisis. Evidence for dyadic accuracy in trait perception—the ability to predict one's interaction partner especially well—has not yet been obtained.

Meta-Perception

Meta-perception refers to perceptions that people have of others' perceptions of them. People grossly overestimate the degree of consistency in how others see them: About 55% of the total variance in meta-perceptions is attributable to the perceiver. Correspondingly, people underestimate how differently others see them: Only about 10% of the variance is attributable to relationship. Virtually none of the variance is at the target level. Perceivers do not consistently see targets as harsh or lenient judges of others.

Meta-accuracy refers to the degree to which meta-perceptions are valid, and is symbolized by $H(Z) = Z(H(Z))$. Meta-perceptions are somewhat accurate in that people do know how others generally see them, assuming that the others agree about the people they are rating. However, people are generally not able to discriminate very well how particular others differentially see them. Common sense suggests that people base their meta-perceptions on how others react to them. Yet the research evidence indicates that people think others see them much as they see themselves. Meta-perception reflects how people see themselves either generally or in the particular interaction.

Self-Perception

Self-perception is marked by self-enhancement: People see themselves more positively than they are seen by others. Interestingly, people show self-abasement in their ratings of Emotional Stability, at least initially. Although there is a general tendency toward self-enhancement, there is also evidence of individual differences: Some people self-enhance more than others do. Once people become acquainted, there is about the same amount of variance in self- and other-perception.

There is strong evidence for assumed similarity; that is, people see others as they see themselves. This is symbolized by $Z(H) = Z(Z)$. The assumed-similarity correlations are about .40. Agreeableness exhibits the greatest level of assumed similarity. The most likely explanation of this result is assumed reciprocity: People assume that because they are agreeable, others will respond in kind.

Contrary to a conclusion drawn by Shrauger and Schoeneman (1979), people see themselves as others do. The self–other agreement correlation, symbolized by $Z(Z) = H(Z)$, is about .40 for most factors and is .70 for Extroversion. However, peers agree more with each other than they agree with the self.

Self-perception is generally, though not always, less valid than other-perception. Others, when given sufficient opportunity to observe a target, more closely estimate the target's actual behavior than the target himself or herself does. This result has very important implications for research in personality. If social scientists are to understand how people differ from one another, they might be better advised to rely on other-perception (peer judgments) more than on self-perceptions. For too long, personality research has relied almost exclusively on self-perception.

Affect

Affect or liking is largely relational: About 40% of the variance in liking is at the level of the relationship. Whom people like is largely idiosyncratic: Perceiver explains about 20% of the variance, and target about 10%.

Affect is closely tied to uniqueness in other-perception, the correlation being about .65. This link is greater if the trait is more inferential and less observable. Moreover, acquaintance appears to result in an increasing correlation between affect and other-perception.

It is well documented that relational attraction is reciprocal and that this dyadic reciprocity increases over time. The dyadic-reciprocity correlation is about .61 when the people are well acquainted and about .26 when they are not so well acquainted. Generalized reciprocity, or the correlation between perceiver and target effects, is not much different from zero for affect.

There is very strong assumed reciprocity of affect at the dyadic level. A person assumes that if he or she likes someone, that someone likes him or her in return. Reciprocity is also assumed at the level of the individual: If someone is liked by others, it is assumed that the person likes others; and if someone likes others, that someone assumes that others like him or her.

Assumed reciprocity of affect also exists in triadic meta-perceptions of affect: If Heidi thinks that Zelda likes Carol, Heidi thinks that Carol likes Zelda.

The Big Five

To make the presentation manageable, the Big Five personality factors have been used to organize the results. There are, however, many other ways to organize personality traits. For instance, traits vary in their scope (Gidron, Koehler, & Tversky, 1993). Traits like "sincere" imply that the person is always sincere, and these have a wide scope, whereas traits like "imaginative" have a more narrow scope. Reeder and Brewer (1979) made a similar distinction. Traits also vary in their observability and evaluative extremity. It would be interesting to answer the nine basic questions by organizing traits in different ways besides the Big Five (see the later section of this chapter on the limits of SRM).

The Big Five cover traits, not emotions or behaviors. It seems likely that judgments of emotions would be much more situational than judgments of traits. Also not considered in this book are athletic ability, physical appearance, and nonverbal skill.

The Puzzling Triangle

Figure 10.1 presents three different components: the person's self-perception, the person's perceiver effect, and the person's target effect.

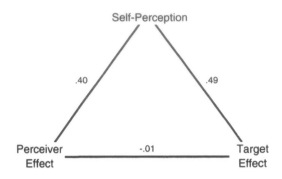

FIGURE 10.1. The puzzling triangle.

Consider the degree of linkage or correlation between each. There is strong evidence for assumed similarity, the correlation between self-perception and the perceiver effect. Using the results in Table 9.4, one obtains an average correlation of *.40*. There is also evidence for self–other agreement: People see themselves as others see them. Using the results in Table 9.7, one obtains an average correlation of *.49*.

Given these two correlations, the expectation is for a modest perceiver–target correlation. The statistical expectation would be for a correlation of .40 × .49, or about .20. However, using the results in Table 6.2, one obtains an average perceiver–target correlation of only *−.01*. The correlations in Figure 10.1 are puzzling: If self-perception correlates with both perceiver and target effects, the expectation is for a perceiver-target correlation. So the virtual absence of such a correlation is odd.

To resolve the puzzle, it can be argued that two different sources bring about the self–perceiver correlation and the self–target correlation. Self-perception may reflect two relatively independent components: an enhancement component and a valid component. The two-component model of self-perception is diagrammed in Figure 10.2. The enhancement component of self-perception creates the self–perceiver correlation. So those who engage in self-enhancement also engage in "other-enhancement"; that is, they differ in how positively they view others. The valid part of self-perception is the part that correlates with the target effect. The model in Figure 10.2 assumes that neither the person's actual standing on the trait nor the target effect directly causes the perceiver effect.

Given this two-component theory of self-perception, it follows that

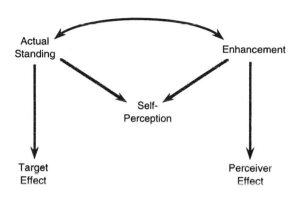

FIGURE 10.2. The two-component model of self-perception.

the perceiver–target correlation reflects the correlation between the valid and enhancement parts of self-perception. The implication of the two-component explanation is that the correlation is rather small because the perceiver–target correlation is so small.

An alternative, but related, view of the puzzling triangle was developed by Malloy (1987b). He called the enhancement component in Figure 10.2 "response set" (see Chapter 3). Malloy also allowed self-perception to cause the perceiver effect, and so he obtained an estimate of assumed similarity. To be able to estimate this causal effect, Malloy (1987b) had to assume that the two components are not correlated. So in Malloy's model, there is a path from self-perception to the perceiver effect, and no correlation between the components.

The major implication of Malloy's model is that to estimate the relationship between self- and other-perception, the perceiver–target correlation should be used. Because the perceiver–target correlations are generally low (see Table 6.2), Malloy (1987b) concluded that there is little or no evidence for assumed similarity.

Interestingly, both Malloy's model and the two-component model view the correlation between self-perception and the perceiver effect as not indicating assumed similarity. The two-component model views the correlation as a reflection that people who engage in self-enhancement also engage in other-enhancement. Malloy views the self–perceiver correlation as a by-product of response set. Based on evidence presented in Chapter 3, it would appear that the perceiver effect is more than response set, and so the two-component model seems more plausible than Malloy's model.

The Weighted-Average Model

A general model of perception, called WAM, has been used to under-stand many of the basic questions. WAM, as presented in Appendix C, has 11 parameters (the nine defined in Chapter 4, plus two additional ones) and can examine how the effects of culture, stereotypes, communication, common ground, and personality mesh to determine perception. Although WAM is a formal model, it has limitations, some of which are discussed in this section. First, however, the relationship between WAM and SRM is reviewed.

The Weighted-Average Model and the Social Relations Model

It is important to understand the differences between WAM and SRM. WAM is a model of how a person perceives another person, and so it is a theoretical model of interpersonal perception. SRM is a model that partitions variance into perceiver, target, and relationship components, and so it is a statistical rather than a theoretical model. WAM and SRM are totally distinct and should not be confused.

If the theoretical model assumed by WAM were true, then that assumption has implications for SRM sources of variance in trait ratings. The parameters within WAM that imply perceiver, target, and relationship effects are discussed.

The perceiver effect is largely represented by the unique impression in WAM. The portion of the unique impression that does not vary across targets can be considered the perceiver effect. Also, a part of the physical-appearance information reveals itself in the perceiver effect. Stereotypes about physical appearance (e.g., sex, age, ethnicity) that are unique to the perceiver and common to all the targets are reflected in the perceiver effect.

As discussed in Chapter 4, the target effect is attributable to several sources: overlap, similar meaning systems, agreement about stereotypes, consistency, and communication. Overlap refers to two perceivers' viewing the same acts. If two perceivers view the same acts and they assign similar meanings to these acts, the perceivers should agree, resulting in a target effect. Also, to the extent to which there is consistency in the target's behaviors, there is going to be a target effect, again if there is some degree of similarity of meaning about the behaviors. Moreover, if perceivers share the same stereotypes about the targets, target effects should emerge. Finally, if the perceivers talk with each other, they are likely to reach some level of agreement.

As discussed in Chapter 5, the relationship effect is attributable to the unique impression, lack of similar meaning systems, and nonoverlap. To the extent to which the perceiver's unique impression varies across targets, dyadic effects are produced. Also, if the same act is given a different meaning, there should be relationship effects. Finally, nonoverlap leads to relationship effects.

Basic Assumptions about Person Perception

WAM makes very strong assumptions about social behavior. It treats person perceivers as "bean counters" or accountants who keep a running total of all the information that they observe. The person perceiver is not seen as an active processor of information.

Consider the role of inconsistency. A perceiver views a target who first helps a friend study for a test and later steals a pack of gum from a convenience store. One act indicates altruism and the other does not. According to WAM, the perceiver merely assigns scale values to each act, adds them, and divides by the sum of the weights. It seems more likely that most perceivers would think of reasons for discounting the importance of one act. For example, the stealing would be rationalized by the claim that the store could afford the loss of a pack of gum. This example points to two weaknesses in WAM: First, some acts are given more weight than other acts; second, the perceiver works hard at developing a consistent integration of the acts.

It seems likely that some key acts play a strong role in the perception of the target and that they are given greater weight in the perceptual process. According to Park, DeKay, and Kraus (1994), it is the unequal weighting that leads to different narrative accounts in perception. That is, the perceiver sees one or two acts as most reflective of a person's personality, and organizes the impression around those acts. Brunswik's (1956) lens model of perception also implies that the cues are differentially weighted by the perceiver.

One important challenge is to mesh WAM's view of interpersonal perception with the view that interpersonal perception is more configural and constructive. The view that perceivers have a mental model (Read & Miller, 1993) of the target needs to be reconciled with WAM. One resolution is to conceive of interpersonal perception in terms of dual processes. Generally, person perception operates according to WAM. But sometimes when salient acts occur or when experimenters ask perceivers to provide accounts, perceivers adopt a more holistic, Gestalt approach to perception.

WAM, as presently conceived, makes no distinction about who is perceiving the target. It would seem that there would be qualitative differences in perception when the perceiver is the partner in the inter-action, the target (i.e., self-perception), or an observer of the interac-tion. Family researchers (e.g., Surra & Ridley, 1991) have speculated extensively on the differences between the perceptions of insiders and outsiders.

The Kernel of Truth in Stereotypes

The version of WAM presented in this book allows for stereotypes based on the physical appearance of the target. It is not too surprising that there is a great deal of agreement about these stereotypes. What is more surprising is that many groups of researchers have found evi-dence that stereotypes have a kernel of truth. In Chapter 7, evidence is presented that judgments made at zero acquaintance (Levesque & Kenny, 1993) have some degree of validity. Also using a variant of the zero-acquaintance paradigm, Borkenau and Liebler (1992) report evidence of the validity of judgments based on minimal information. Finally, Berry (1990) reports evidence that judgments based on pho-tographs have surprising validity. Ambady and Rosenthal (1992), in a meta-analysis of 44 studies, have argued that "thin slices" of behavior lead to surprising accuracy. Quite clearly, there is good reason to sup-pose that there is a kernel of truth in some stereotypes about physical appearance.

Bigots should not take any comfort in these conclusions. First, the evidence is not that all stereotypes are valid. In particular, there is little or no evidence that racial and sexual stereotypes have any va-lidity in person perception. Second, stereotypes sometimes create their own reality via the self-fulfilling prophecy (to be discussed later in this chapter). So a stereotype may be true only because people believe that it is true.

Summary

Although WAM has some severe limitations, it does allow for the simul-taneous operation of 11 different parameters and predicts consensus and accuracy. In Chapter 9, a method is outlined to allow WAM to explain self–other agreement. Moreover, unlike other models, WAM permits communication effects. Despite its limitations, WAM is a powerful tool for understanding interpersonal perception.

The Social Relations Model

SRM has proved to be a useful vehicle in the understanding of interpersonal perception. But like any tool, it does have limitations, and some of them are considered in this section.

Limitations

Perhaps the major limitation is that the statistics and data analysis of the model are complicated. Within psychology, the dominant way of treating data is to compute means and compare those means by an analysis of variance. A researcher using SRM computes not means, but variances and correlations. These are not even the usual variances and correlations, in that they are inferred statistics and not directly computed (see Chapter 2). They are so unusual that the variances can be negative and the correlations can be larger than 1. Thus, SRM requires a very new way of thinking about data analysis.

Because these complicated statistics are nonstandard, basic statistical packages cannot be used, and so specialized computer software must be developed. Computer programs have been written (Kenny, 1993a, 1993b), but they have limited distribution at present. Ideally, in the future the computer programs will become more widely accessible and will be available in standard packages.

One considerable limitation of SRM is the design requirement of multiple interactions with multiple partners. Moreover, these interactions must be structured in very systematic ways (i.e., block or round-robin). Even when a complicated design is used, missing data present such a problem that the loss of just one data point may require the loss of an entire group. The requirement of multiple partners makes the study of close relationships more difficult. Very little of the research reviewed in this book concerns people in close, long-term relationships. It is no accident that in all too many of the studies employed here, the subjects began as totally unacquainted. Of the over 50 published papers using SRM to date, only about 5 concern married couples.

Although SRM is a helpful tool that can be used to understand perception and behavior, it is not itself a theory of interpersonal behavior. Nonetheless, by partitioning the variance, it points to the major sources of variance and level at which the behavior and perceptions operate. SRM explicitly recognizes two levels of analysis: the person and the dyad.

Future Research

What questions can SRM easily answer, and what questions pose difficulties for the model? First, the model can directly answer the nine basic questions posed in Chapter 1. From Chapters 3 to 9, SRM has been used to determine the existence of consensus, assimilation, meta-accuracy, and the like. Moreover, for many questions, the model differentiates the questions at two levels: the person and the relationship.

The model can directly examine questions about correlates of components. So if one has a measure that is supposed to correlate with interpersonal perceptions, that measure can be correlated with those perceptions. However, the text has not extensively explored this type of hypothesis. The one major exception is for the correlation between the perceiver effect in meta-perception and various personality measures (see Table 8.6), where it has been found that the perceiver effect in meta-perception correlates with social anxiety and need for social approval.

Numerous hypotheses about correlates of the components deserve investigation. Here are a few examples:

Do men or women have more positive perceiver effects?
If the perceiver and target are involved in a close relationship, does the perceiver view the target more favorably?
If the target is physically attractive, is he or she liked more?

There is one class of hypotheses that the model has difficulty handling: moderators of the basic questions. A "moderator" is a variable for which the basic interpersonal phenomenon differs. The analysis of moderators is critical for a complete understanding of interpersonal perception (Paunonen, 1989; Paunonen & Jackson, 1985). Below are examples of four types of moderators:

1. Do people show greater consensus when they are rating male or female targets?
2. Are depressives less likely to assume similarity?
3. Are people more accurate when they are rating someone to whom they feel close?
4. Is there more reciprocity in ratings of Agreeableness than of Extroversion?

Moderators can be classified as person moderators (e.g., perceiver or target), relational moderators, and trait moderators. The first two questions are examples of person moderators, the first being a target moderator and the second being a perceiver moderator. The third question is an example of a relational moderator, and the fourth question is an example of a trait moderator.

SRM can most easily handle trait moderators. Consider the moderation of consensus. Each trait is analyzed separately, and the level of consensus is compared. The Big Five factors have been treated as trait moderators throughout the book. Sometimes relational moderators can be treated as trait moderators. For example, acquaintance, which is fundamentally a relational variable, is often treated as a trait moderator. That is, the same people are studied when they are relatively unacquainted and later when they are more acquainted.

Categorical person moderators (e.g., sex) can be studied within SRM in one of three ways (Malloy & Kenny, 1986). Consider the person moderator of sex. The first way is to form homogeneous groups (i.e., males judging males and females judging females). Consensus can be compared for the two groups. If there is more consensus in the female group, there are two alternate explanations: Females as perceivers show more consensus, or females as targets create more consensus.

Alternatively, heterogeneous groups can be formed (i.e., males judging females and females judging males). If there is more consensus when females judge males, there are again two alternate explanations. In an ideal study, all possible groups are formed: males judging males, males judging females, females judging males, and females judging males. Such a study can be accomplished by a block–round-robin design (Kenny, 1990) in which there are at least four males and four females.

If the person moderators are continuous variables (e.g., age or depression), the strategy of creating discrete groups is usually not feasible. So, for instance, there are no SRM analyses of the "depressive realism" hypothesis. Continuous variables such as depression can be studied by allowing for differential sensitivity, as discussed in Chapter 5. Differential sensitivity measures which perceivers are more sensitive to the stimulus information. Currently there is no standard analysis strategy for measuring and testing differential sensitivity, but I hope that one will be developed soon.

Relational moderators are the most difficult type of moderators to study within SRM. Because relational variables such as similarity, closeness, and liking are critical variables in the understanding of interpersonal perception, it is unfortunate that they cannot be easily studied.

Consider the measurement of consensus as a function of closeness. One strategy, outlined elsewhere (Kenny & Albright, 1987), is to measure the agreement for each dyad. To do this, one begins with an SRM design (i.e., round-robin), and each perceiver rates the target on a series of traits. A correlation or some other measure of association is computed for each perceiver–target combination across the set of traits. Then this measure of association is analyzed by SRM. It is determined whether consensus correlates with closeness at the relationship level. I hope that this and c .her methods of studying relational moderators will be explored.

The Notational System

One useful feature of this book is that it has presented a simple notational system for perception, meta-perception, and self-perception, which was originally developed a few years ago (Kenny, 1988). Heidi's perception of Zelda is denoted as $H(Z)$; how Zelda thinks Heidi sees her is denoted as $Z(H(Z))$; and Heidi's self-perception is denoted as $H(H)$. The basic questions in interpersonal perception can be simply and elegantly expressed using this notation. So, for instance, assumed reciprocity is symbolized by $Z(H) = Z(H(Z))$.

In this book, Zelda's perceiver effect is denoted as $Z(\text{\textdagger})$ and Zelda's target effect as $\text{\textdagger}(Z)$. The unique perception that Zelda has of Heidi is denoted as $z(h)$. With this notation, many of the basic questions can be expressed at two levels. So, for instance, reciprocity at the individual level is expressed as $Z(\text{\textdagger}) = \text{\textdagger}(Z)$, and reciprocity at the dyadic level is given as $z(h) = h(z)$.

Nine basic questions have been proposed in Chapter 1 and translated into SRM terms in Chapter 2. In Chapter 8, a new question has been introduced: Does Zelda think that others see her as she sees herself, or $Z(\text{\textdagger}(Z)) = Z(Z)$? This question might be called assumed similarity between self- and meta-perception.

Except only briefly in Chapter 6, this book has not examined triadic perceptions. Meta-perception is a fundamentally triadic process: Zelda may wonder how Heidi views Carol, or, in the notation, $Z(H(C))$. However, in this book the meta-perceptions are always dyadic: How does Zelda think that Heidi sees her? Recently, two studies (Chapdelaine, Kenny, & LaFontana, in press; Frey & Smith, 1993) have examined the triadic meta-perception of liking. Moreover, social network researchers (Krackhardt, 1987) have become interested in cognitive social structures that are triadic. A full examination of triadic processes requires an extension of SRM to allow for three, not two, factors.

Several interesting questions can be addressed at the triadic level. Among them are assumed reciprocity, or $Z(H(C)) = Z(C(H))$, and meta-accuracy, or $H(C) = Z(H(C))$. Also, do people know how others see themselves, or $Z(H(H)) = H(H)$? Future work will investigate these fascinating triadic phenomena. However, SRM will first have to be expanded to consider a third person.

Moving beyond the triadic level does not really seem necessary. Although Laing, Phillipson, and Lee (1966) consider such questions, it seems that for the moment the field of interpersonal perception can be kept busy enough studying dyadic and triadic phenomena.

The notation could also be extended to include the trait being perceived. So Zelda's perception of Heidi's Culture could be symbolized as $Z(H_V)$, where the "V" refers to Factor V of the Big Five. By convention, the trait symbol would be placed on the innermost term. So the meta-perception of Agreeableness (Factor II) would be symbolized by $Z(H(Z_{II}))$.

The notation could also be used to denote classes of targets or perceivers. For instance, M_1 and M_2 might denote male perceivers, and F_1 and F_2 female perceivers. So the statement

$$[F_1(Z) = F_2(Z)] > [M_1(Z) = M_2(Z)]$$

would imply that female perceivers exhibit more consensus than male perceivers.

The major value of the notation is that it takes very complicated statements (e.g., if John thinks Mary is intelligent, does Mary think that John thinks she is intelligent?) and condenses them into a simple, interpretable expression [i.e., $J(M) = M(J(M))$].

Behavior and Perception

The major topic of this book is perception: How do people see others, how do people see themselves, and how do people think others see them? But at various times (especially during the discussion of target accuracy in Chapter 7), there has been a consideration of the relationship between perception and behavior.

In this section, I explore in more detail the links between perception and behavior. First considered are the ways in which behavior determines perception (e.g., accuracy) at the level of the individual. I then consider the ways in which perception determines behavior (e.g., the self-fulfilling prophecy), again at the individual level. Next, linkages between behavior and perception are explored at the dyadic level. Finally, I discuss the design and analysis of behavioral studies.

Not explored in this section is the relationship between meta-perception and behavior. These effects probably exist and may be very important. For instance, people may alter their behavior because they think that someone sees them in a particular way.

Assume that there is a group of people, all of whom interact dyadically with each other. The friendliness of each person's behavior is measured, ignoring all the complications in the measurement of behavior that have been discussed in Chapter 7. Also people are asked both how friendly their interaction partners are and how friendly they see themselves as being across all their interactions. So measures of behavior and perception are obtained. When reference to a particular person is needed, I use the person Kerry, a member of the group.

Effects from Behavior to Perceptions

Behavior is partitioned into actor, partner, and relationship effects. The term $K_\uparrow$ represents the level at which an actor named Kerry tends to behave with all of her interaction partners. So if Kerry has a positive actor effect, she tends to be friendly with her interaction partners. The partner effect in behavior, or $\uparrow_K$, is the behavior that Kerry tends to elicit from others. So for friendliness, $\uparrow_K$ refers to the tendency of Kerry to "make" others act friendly when they interact with her.

The impressions that people have of each other can also be partitioned into Perceiver or $K(\uparrow)$ and Target or $\uparrow(K)$. As it has been throughout this text, the perceiver effect represents how the person generally sees others, and the target effect represents how the person is generally seen by others. Finally, there is the person's self-perception, or $K(K)$.

There are other factors besides behavior that cause perceptions. So for Perceiver, Target, and Self, there are residual or disturbance sources of variance. For Perceiver, the set of residual causes is designated as Q, which represents the stereotype that the person has of the group. For Target, the other causes are designated as U, which includes all other causes of perception that are not attributable to the person's behavior. So the term U represents the consistent biases in social perception. For instance, if a culture has sex-role stereotypes that are false, they are reflected in U. Finally, for Self, the disturbance is designated as E, which represents bias or error in self-perception. It measures the degree to which some individuals self-enhance more than others. These terms and their definitions are presented in Table 10.1.

So there are two exogenous or causal factors, the Actor and the Partner, for behavior; three endogenous or effect variables, Perceiver, Target, and Self; and disturbance or residual term for each endogenous

TABLE 10.1. List of Causes and Effects in the Model of How Behavior Determines Perception at the Individual Level

Causes

Actor	How friendly the person is across interaction partners
Partner	How friendly the person's interaction partners are

Effects

Perceiver	How friendly the person sees others
Target	How friendly the person is seen by others
Self	How friendly the person sees self

Disturbances (other causes)

Q	View of the typical other; group stereotype
U	Mistakes made in the target effect (e.g., sex-role stereotypes)
E	Mistakes made in self-perception; self-enhancement

variable, Q, U, and E. The causal model of the effects from behavior to perception is presented in Figure 10.3.

All the causal links are listed in Table 10.2. First considered are the effects on the Perceiver variable, or how the person tends to view others. A person's view of others can be attributed to the behavior of others with whom he or she interacts. If all of a person's interaction partners tend to be friendly, and the person sees his or her partners as friendly, the person is accurate. This form of accuracy is called "perceiver accuracy" in Chapter 7.

The person's view of others may be colored by his or her own behavior. A person who is friendly may tend to see others as friendly.

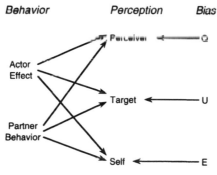

FIGURE 10.3. Effects of behavior on perception at the individual level.

TABLE 10.2. Model of the Effects from Behavior to Perception

Effect	Cause	Interpretation
Perceiver	Partner	Perceiver accuracy
	Actor	Perceiver misattribution
	Q	Group stereotype
Target	Actor	Target accuracy
	Partner	Target misattribution
	U	Bias in perception
Self	Actor	Self-accuracy
	Partner	Self-misattribution
	E	Self-enhancement

This is a form of misattribution, in that the person attributes his or her own friendliness to the partner. Finally, there are the other causes of the Perceiver effect, which are represented by Q (the stereotype that the perceiver has of the group members being rated).

The Target effect may be caused by the Actor effect in behavior. This has been called "target accuracy" in Chapter 7. A person who behaves in a friendly manner is seen by his or her partners as friendly.

The Target effect may also be caused by the Partner effect in behavior. This effect can be described as misattribution: The behavior of the person's interaction partners causes the perception of him or her. So if Kerry's interaction partners are friendly, she is seen as friendly, controlling for the level of friendliness in her behavior. Finally, there are biases in person perception, represented by U. Stereotypes based on physical appearance are included in this term.

Self-perception is caused by behavior. How people see themselves is presumably attributable to how they behave. So the path from the Actor effect to Self-perception represents accuracy.

The path from Partner to Self-perception represents misattribution: If a person "makes" others friendly, he or she may see himself or herself as friendly. Finally, there are errors in self-perception, represented by the variable E (which largely represents self-enhancement).

The disturbances of the Perceiver, Target, and Self variables are probably correlated. The correlation between Q and U may be attributable to some physical characteristic of the target. For instance, it may be that the gender of the target leads to stereotypes (reflected in U), and that gender also leads to biases in perception (reflected in Q). The correlation between Q and E can be interpreted in terms of processes discussed earlier in this chapter: People who engage in self-enhancement also engage in other-enhancement. The correlation between U and E can be interpreted as the degree to which self-enhancement leads to bias in the perception of the target. So if the person has an inflated view of himself or herself, others have an inflated view of him or her.

In summary, it is interesting to note that Perceiver, Target, and Self all have three different sets of causes. There is one set that represents accuracy, another that represents misattribution, and a third set that represents errors in perception. Misattribution is different from other errors in that it is based on behavior, but it is based on the "wrong" person's behavior.

Self-Fulfilling Prophecy Effects

Work in social science has long emphasized the role that perceptions play in creating their own reality. Starting with the pioneering work of Merton (1957), and continuing through the landmark efforts of Rosenthal (1966) on expectancy effects and the work by Snyder and Swann (1978) on behavioral confirmation, the self-fulfilling prophecy is a cornerstone of social science theorizing. In a review of the evidence on self-fulfilling prophecy, Jussim (1991) has argued that behavior may be more a cause than a consequence of perception. However, Jussim acknowledges the effect that perception has on behavior.

In this section, the causation goes from perception to behavior: People alter their behavior to conform to the perception that others and they themselves have. I examine how Perceiver, Target, and Self influence the Actor and Partner effects in behavior. These six possible effects are listed in Table 10.3.

Considered first are the influences on the Actor effect, or how a person behaves across his or her interaction partners. The example

TABLE 10.3. Model of the Effects from Perception to Behavior

Effect	Cause	Interpretation
Actor	Perceiver	Perceiver complementary projection
	Target	Target self-fulfilling prophecy
	Self	Self-actualization
Partner	Perceiver	Perceiver self-fulfilling prophecy
	Target	Target complementary projection
	Self	Other-actualization

to be discussed, again, is the friendliness of a person named Kerry. The effect from Perceiver to Actor is a case of complementary projection (discussed in Chapter 6): Kerry's way of seeing others makes her change her behavior. So, if Kerry thinks that others are friendly, she behaves in a friendly fashion. She adopts a behavioral style consistent with her expectations.

The effect from Target to Actor is the classical self-fulfilling prophecy: If people see a target in a certain way, that target behaves in a way consistent with the perception. For instance, if others think that Kerry is a friendly person, this perception leads Kerry to become a friendly person. Probably this effect, if it exists, is mediated by the Partner effect in behavior. Others think that Kerry is friendly; they behave in a friendly way with Kerry; and this produces friendliness in Kerry.

The final influence on the Actor is from the Self. That is, expectations or perceptions about the self lead to changes in behavior. Kerry sees herself as a friendly person, and this leads her to act as a friendly person. This effect is called here "self-actualization," a central concept in Maslow's (1954) humanistic psychology. Swann's (1990) self-verification theory also predicts causal effects from self-perception to behavior.

Considered now are the influences on the Partner effect in behavior: how Kerry "makes" others behave. So, for example, when people are with Kerry, they behave in a more friendly manner than they would otherwise. The Perceiver effect may influence the Partner effect: Kerry, who tends to view others as friendly, "makes" other behave in a friendly fashion. This is a self-fulfilling prophecy, but in this case the effect is from Perceiver to Partner, whereas the classical self-fulfilling prophecy effect is from Target to Actor. It seems likely that this effect, if it exists, is mediated by the Actor effect in behavior. That is, if Kerry thinks that others are friendly, she then behaves in a friendly manner, and this behavior leads to friendly behavior in others.

The Target effect in perception may influence the Partner effect in behavior. How others evaluate a target may change how others behave with the target. So if people think that Kerry is friendly, they may act in a friendly fashion when interacting with Kerry. This is a form of complementary projection: People alter their behavior to conform to their expectations.

Self-perception may also influence the Partner effect in behavior. Kerry, who sees herself as friendly, makes others behave as friendly. This is called "other-actualization," because in this case self-perception changes not the self but others. It seems likely that this effect, if it exists, is mediated by the Actor effect in behavior. That is, if Kerry thinks that she is friendly, she then behaves in a friendly manner, and this behavior leads to friendly behavior in others.

Dyadic Behavior–Perception Linkages

The preceding sections have considered the links between perception and behavior at the level of the individual. In this section, the effects of perception on behavior and the effects of behavior on perception at the level of relationship are considered.

There are four effects that describe the potential linkages between perception and behavior at the dyadic level. Table 10.4 presents them in a 2 × 2 table. They involve the two types of dyadic effects, intrapersonal and interpersonal (see Chapter 2), and the effects from behavior to perception and from perception to behavior. The effect names are taken from the preceding two sections.

Consider the interaction between Zelda and Heidi in which friendliness is measured. The intrapersonal effect from behavior to perception is a misattribution. If Zelda behaves in friendly fashion, she sees Heidi as friendly. The interpersonal effect from behavior to perception is dyadic accuracy. If Zelda behaves in a friendly fashion with Heidi, Heidi sees Zelda as a friendly person.

The effects from perception to behavior are as follows: The intrapersonal effect is a form of complementary projection. If Zelda sees Heidi as friendly, Zelda behaves in a friendly manner with Heidi. The interpersonal effect is the dyadic self-fulfilling prophecy. If Zelda perceives Heidi as friendly, Heidi acts friendly when interacting with Zelda.

The Design and Analysis of Behavioral Observations

Some guidance on the design of behavioral studies may be helpful. One key question is the timing of the measurement of behavior in relation to the measurement of perception. Sometimes the behavior of the targets is measured before the perceivers observe and rate the targets; in this case, the research question is how behavior determines perception.

TABLE 10.4. Model of Relationship Effects

Direction of effect	Intrapersonal	Interpersonal
Behavior to perception	Misattribution	Accuracy
Perception to behavior	Complementary projection	Self-fulfilling prophecy

Alternatively, the perception is measured before behavior; this type of design reveals how well perception can be used to predict behavior.

Another key issue is whether the perceivers directly observe the behavior that is coded before the perceivers make their judgments. If they do, then the study concerns how behavior determines perception. If they do not, the study is one of predictive accuracy. Also, if the interest is in the self-fulfilling prophecy, the perception should be measured before the behavior.

Who are the raters? Normally, the raters or coders of behavior are different people from the perceivers and targets. If the perceivers or targets are used to measure behavior, there may be large expectancy effects. So the data structure for behavioral observations is generally triadic: raters evaluating dyadic interactions. Typically, there are very few raters, and results are simply averaged across the raters (once interrater reliability is demonstrated); thus raters are ignored in the analysis. If the raters observe all of the interactions, they can be treated as variables, and their reliability in judging perceiver, target, and relationship can be ascertained. The reader is urged to review the section on behavioral observation in Chapter 7, which details guidelines on the measurement of the reliability from behavioral observations.

What is known about the variance partitioning of behavioral data? Unfortunately, not many SRM studies have examined behavior. However, a rough working rule of thumb, based on prior empirical work (Dabbs & Ruback, 1987; Kenny & Malloy, 1988; Levesque & Kenny, 1993; Ross & Lollis, 1989; Warner, Kenny, & Stoto, 1979), is a "35-0-15-50" rule: 35% actor effects, no partner effects, 15% relationship effects, and 50% error.

Some readers may be surprised that as much as 35% of the variance in behavior is attributable to the actor. Behavior is, in fact, consistent from partner to partner. If there is consistency in people's behavior, it can be asked why consensus is so low. Perhaps in forming perceptions about others, people use the relationship effect in behavior in forming impressions. That is, Heidi's perception of Zelda is more influenced by Zelda's behavioral relationship effect than by Zelda's behavioral actor effect. Such an effect would imply that perceivers are sensitive to how they are differentially treated by targets.

Partner effects in behavior are more elusive. In our most extensive search for them (Kenny & Malloy, 1988), we found little or no evidence for them. If there are weak partner effects in behavior, the models discussed earlier become much simpler, in that many effects can be set to zero.

There has been very little work on relationship effects and behavior. Ross and Lollis (1989) have written an important paper arguing that relationship effects in behavior should be used as an index of whether people are relating to each other. The amount of relationship variance should change, depending on the type of behavior under study. To use a trivial example, if kissing is the behavior, there is likely to be much greater relationship variance and much less actor variance.

Reciprocity of behavior, particularly nonverbal behavior, has long been a subject of considerable interest (Cappella, 1981). However, reciprocity has generally been more commonly used in the *temporal* sense of the term (Zelda smiles at Heidi, and then Heidi smiles at Zelda) than in the *dyadic* sense of the term (Zelda is especially likely to smile at Heidi, and Heidi is especially likely to smile at Zelda). Presumably, there is reciprocity of prosocial and antisocial behaviors. It is known that who speaks to whom in groups is reciprocal, and that it is more reciprocal in socioemotional than in task-oriented groups (Dabbs & Ruback, 1987). However, a full-scale investigation of reciprocity of behavior within SRM has yet to be completed.

Postscript

The application of SRM to the study of interpersonal perception has led to many important insights. It has made what seems like a simple and straightforward topic much more complicated than common sense would suggest. But these complications are essential. The partitioning of social perception into components may seem to some an unnecessary waste of time. There were some who objected to separating the atom into protons, neutrons, and electrons, which in turn were later divided into quarks. If the understanding of physical matter requires the analysis of unobservable components, it should not surprise us that for a full understanding of interpersonal perception, there must be a separation into components.

There are some serious limitations in the investigation. Virtually all of the research to date has used college students. Not enough of the research has employed children, and virtually none of the studies have used people over 40 years of age. Also with few exceptions, the research participants have been white middle-class people from the United States. Finally, as previously stated, the traits have been organized by the Big Five, and other ways of organizing the traits have not been given much attention.

This investigation of interpersonal perception has been completed. Our journey has now come to an end. Much has been learned, but much still remains to be discovered. I hope that this book will stimulate interest into these most important questions. I invite the reader to partake in this most exciting intellectual adventure.

STUDY DESCRIPTIONS

W hat follows is a brief description of the studies that are reviewed in various chapters. Included are only studies to which I have access for SRM analyses. For each study, the following is presented:

The number of perceivers.
The average number of targets per perceiver (the range is given if this number varies).
The number of trait, affect, or other measures at each time point.
The number of time points or waves (if there is just 1, this is omitted).
The degree of acquaintance between judges and targets.
The setting of the research.
The type of task (if the setting is the laboratory).
The type of research design.
What secondary sources used the data, if any.[1]
The chapters of this book in which results are presented.

Albright (1990): 67 perceivers; 4.58 targets per perceiver (4 to 8); 5 traits; 3 waves; zero and short-term group; residential; round-robin; discussed in Chapters 4 and 9.

Albright, Kenny, & Malloy (1988), Study 1: 42 perceivers; 3.67 targets per perceiver (3 to 4); 5 traits; 3 waves; zero and short-term group; classroom; round-robin; only wave 1 presented in the article and 15 people lost over time; discussed in Chapters 4, 5, 6, and 9.

Albright, Kenny, & Malloy (1988), Study 2: 33 perceivers; 3.76 targets per perceiver (3 to 4); 5 traits; zero; classroom; round-robin; discussed in Chapters 4 and 9.

Parts of this appendix are adapted from Kenny, Albright, Malloy, and Kashy (in press). Copyright 1994 by the American Psychological Association. Adapted by permission.

Albright, Kenny, & Malloy (1988), Study 3: 169 perceivers; 3.76 targets per perceiver (3 to 5); 10 traits; zero; classroom; round-robin; discussed in Chapters 3, 4, 5, and 9.

Albright-Malloy (1988): 60 perceivers; 3.61 targets per perceiver (3 to 4); 5 traits; 3 waves; long-term; classroom; round-robin; discussed in Chapters 4, 5, and 9.

Anderson (1985): 121 perceivers; 23.1 targets per perceiver (15 to 30); 4 traits; long-term; residential; round-robin; discussed in Chapters 4, 6, and 8.

Bernard, Killworth, & Sailer (1982), Fraternity: 57 perceivers; 56 targets per perceiver; frequency of interaction; long-term; residential; round-robin; used by Kashy and Kenny (1990a); discussed in Chapter 7.

Bernard, Killworth, & Sailer (1982), Ham Radio Operators: 44 perceivers; 43 targets per perceiver; frequency of interaction; long-term; radio communication setting; round-robin; used by Kashy and Kenny (1990a); discussed in Chapter 7.

Bernard, Killworth, & Sailer (1982), Office Workers: 44 perceivers; 43 targets per perceiver; frequency of interaction; long-term; work setting; round-robin; used by Kashy and Kenny (1990a); discussed in Chapter 7.

Bernard, Killworth, & Sailer (1982), Technical Students: 34 perceivers; 33 targets per perceiver; frequency of interaction; long-term; educational setting; round-robin data; used by Kashy and Kenny (1990a); discussed in Chapter 7.

Campbell, Miller, Lubetsky, & O'Connell (1964): 313 perceivers; 18.56 targets per perceiver (7 to 23); 18 traits; long-term; residential; dyad–round-robin; data used by Kenny and Kashy (in press); discussed in Chapters 3, 4, and 6.

Chapdelaine, Kenny, & LaFontana (in press): 120 perceivers; 4 targets per perceiver; 10 traits and 2 measures of affect; short-term one-on-one; laboratory; getting acquainted to make predictions; round-robin; discussed in Chapters 3, 5, and 6.

Curry & Emerson (1970): 48 perceivers; 7 targets per perceiver; liking and perceived liking; 5 waves; long-term; residential; round-robin; data used in Kenny & Nasby (1980) and Kenny & La-Voie (1982); discussed in Chapters 5, 6, and 8.

Dabbs & Ruback (1987): 310 perceivers; 4 targets per perceiver; 2 affect measures; short-term group; laboratory; problem solving and getting acquainted; round-robin; discussed in Chapters 4, 5, 6, and 10.

Dantchik (1985): 60 perceivers; 3.62 targets per perceiver (3 to 4); 6 traits; long-term; residential; round-robin; discussed in Chapters 3, 4, 6, and 9.

DePaulo, Kenny, Hoover, Webb, & Oliver (1987): 42 perceivers; 3 targets per perceiver; 5 traits; 4 waves; short-term one-on-one; laboratory; problem solving; block; discussed in Chapters 4, 5, 6, and 8.

DiPilato (1990): 96 perceivers; 3 targets per perceiver; 10 traits; 2 waves; zero and short-term group; laboratory; problem solving and getting acquainted; round-robin; discussed in Chapters 4 and 9.

Hallmark (1991): 144 perceivers; 2 targets per perceiver; 4 traits; short-term group; laboratory; question and answer; round-robin; discussed in Chapter 4.

Hallmark & Kenny (1989): 163 perceivers; 4.43 targets per perceiver (4 to 5); 6 traits; short-term group; laboratory; problem solving; round-robin; discussed in Chapters 2, 3, 4, 5, and 6.

Kashy (1988): 136 perceivers; 7 targets per perceiver; 1 trait; short-term group; laboratory; competitive trivia task with four against four; block–round-robin; discussed in Chapters 3, 4, 5, and 6.

Kenny (1992): 84 perceivers; 3.94 targets per perceiver (3 to 4); 10 traits; zero; classroom; round-robin; discussed in Chapters 4 and 9.

Kenny & Bernstein (1982): 120 perceivers; 2 targets per perceiver; 4 traits; short-term one-on-one; laboratory; mock date; block; discussed in Chapters 4, 5, and 6.

Kenny & DePaulo (1990), Applicant: 48 perceivers; 3 targets per perceiver; 6 traits; 3 waves; short-term group; laboratory; 3 interviewers questioning an applicant for a residential assistant position; block; discussed in Chapters 4, 5, 6, and 8.

Kenny & DePaulo (1990), Interviewer: 48 perceivers; 3 targets per perceiver; 6 traits; 3 waves; short-term one-on-one; laboratory; as above; block; discussed in Chapters 4, 6, and 8.

Kenny, Horner, Kashy, & Chu (1992), Study 1: 113 perceivers; 32 targets per perceiver; 10 traits; zero; laboratory; videotape judgment; half-block; discussed in Chapters 4 and 9.

Kenny, Horner, Kashy, & Chu (1992), Study 2: 108 perceivers; 3 targets per perceiver; 10 traits; 2 waves; zero and short-term one-on-one; laboratory; getting acquainted; round-robin; discussed in Chapters 3, 4, 5, and 9.

Kenny, Horner, Kashy, & Chu (1992), Study 3: 70 perceivers; 3.26 targets per perceiver (2 to 4); 10 traits; 2 waves; zero and short-term group; classroom; round-robin; discussed in Chapters 4, 5, and 9.

Latané (1987): 68 perceivers; 3 targets per perceiver; 3 traits; zero; laboratory; photograph judgments; round-robin; discussed in Chapters 4 and 9.

Levesque (1990): 142 perceivers; 4.46 targets per perceiver (3 to 5); 7 traits; short-term group; laboratory; mock jury deliberation; round-robin; discussed in Chapters 3, 4, 5, 6, and 9.

Levesque & Kenny (1993): 80 perceivers; 3 targets per perceiver; 17

traits; zero and short-term one-on-one; laboratory; predictions followed by interactions; round-robin; discussed in Chapters 7, 9, and 10.

Levine & Snyder (1980): 50 perceivers; 24 targets per perceiver; 3 measures of affect; long-term; classroom; round-robin; discussed in Chapter 2.

Malloy (1987a): 40 perceivers; 3.44 targets per perceiver (3 to 4); 10 traits; 3 waves; zero and short-term group; classroom; round-robin; 24% of the subjects from Study 3 of Albright et al. (1988); discussed in Chapters 3, 4, and 9.

Malloy & Albright (1990): 68 perceivers; 3 targets per perceiver; 5 traits; long-term; residential; round-robin; discussed in Chapters 4, 5, 6, 8, and 9.

Malloy & Janowski (1992): 68 perceivers; 5.80 targets per perceiver (5 to 7); leadership and meta-perceptions of leadership; short-term group; laboratory; group discussions to consensus; round-robin; discussed in Chapters 5, 6, and 8.

McGillan (1980): 80 perceivers; 2 targets per perceiver; 2 traits; short-term one-on-one; laboratory; getting acquainted; block; discussed in Chapter 4.

Montgomery (1984): 128 perceivers; 3.41 targets per perceiver (3 to 4); 2 traits; 3 waves; short-term group; classroom; round-robin; discussed in Chapters 3, 4, 5, and 9.

Newcomb (1961): 17 perceivers; 16 targets per perceiver; 1 measure of affect; 14 waves; long-term group; residential; round-robin; discussed in Chapters 5 and 6.

Oliver (1989): 56 perceivers; 2 targets per perceiver; 11 traits; short-term one-on-one; laboratory; mock date; block; discussed in Chapters 4, 6, 8, and 9.

Park & Judd (1989), Study 1: 71 perceivers; 7.88 targets per perceiver (6 to 9); 14 traits; 4 waves; short-term group; laboratory; question and answer; round-robin; data used by Park & Flink (1989); discussed in Chapters 3, 4, 5, 6, and 9.

Reno & Kenny (1992): 102 perceivers; 4.1 targets per perceiver (3 to 5); 16 traits; short-term one-on-one; laboratory; getting acquainted; round-robin; discussed in Chapters 4, 6, and 8.

Rothbart & Singer (1988): 78 perceivers; 5 targets per perceiver; 15 traits; short-term group; laboratory; minimal group; round-robin; discussed in Chapters 4 and 6.

Shechtman & Kenny (in press); 154 perceivers; 6.00 targets per perceiver (4 to 9); 4 traits; short-term group; teacher training groups; round-robin; data used by Shechtman (1994); discussed in Chapters 2, 5, 6, 8, and 9.

Schill & Thomsen (1987): 64 perceivers; 2 targets per perceiver; 8 traits; 2 waves; short-term one-on-one; laboratory; competitive discussion; circle; discussed in Chapter 4.

Yingling (1989): 24 perceivers; 3 targets per perceiver; 1 trait; short-term one-on-one; laboratory; getting acquainted; round-robin; discussed in Chapter 4.

Zaccaro, Foti, & Kenny (1991): 108 perceivers; 2 targets per perceiver; rating and ranking of leadership; short-term group; laboratory; work tasks; rotation; discussed in Chapter 3.

Notes

1. However, if Kenny and DePaulo (1993) or Kenny, Albright, Malloy, and Kashy (in press) used the data set, that is not noted because the entire list of studies is presented in Chapters 4 and 8 (see Tables 4.1 and 8.1).

STATISTICAL DETAILS
OF THE SOCIAL
RELATIONS MODEL

I n this appendix, the statistical details for the estimation and testing of variances and correlations from the Social Relations Model (SRM) are presented. First considered is the estimation of single-variable or univariate models. The next topic is the measurement of bivariate correlations in SRM. Last discussed is the estimation of construct variance, which allows for the separation of relationship and error variance. For each of these topics, the analysis of the half-block design, the full-block design, and the round-robin design is presented.

Formally, SRM is as follows for perceiver i rating target j:

$$X_{ij} = m + a_i + b_j + g_{ij}$$

The terms a, b, and g are all random variables with zero mean and variances of σ_a^2, σ_b^2, and σ_g^2. Estimates of these variances are denoted s_a^2, s_b^2, and s_g^2, respectively. There are two nonzero covariances in the model: the perceiver–target covariance, σ_{ab}, and the relationship covariance, $\sigma_{gg'}$. The perceiver–target covariance is between a_i and b_i, and the relationship covariance is between g_{ij} and g_{ji}. The estimates of these covariances are denoted as s_{ab} and $s_{gg'}$. All other covariances are assumed to equal zero.

Traditionally within SRM, estimates are computed for each group of observations (e.g., round-robin or block). With such an estimation approach, the constant may vary across groups, because estimates are computed across groups. We (Kashy & Kenny, 1990b) discuss an alternate estimation procedure that assumes that the constant is the same for each group.

Estimation of Univariate Model

Half-Block Design

Considered first is the estimation for the half-block design. In this design, there are n perceivers and r targets; the perceivers do not serve as targets, and the targets do not serve as perceivers. The half-block design is considered first because its analysis closely resembles an analysis of variance. Denote $M_{i.}$ as the mean rating for perceiver i across the r targets, $M_{.j}$ as the mean rating for target j across the n perceivers, and $M_{..}$ as the mean rating across all rn judgments. The estimates of perceiver, target, and relationship effects are as follows. Person i's estimated perceiver effect is

$$\hat{a}_i = M_{i.} - M_{..}$$

The estimate of person j's target effect is

$$\hat{b}_j = M_{.j} - M_{..}$$

The estimate of the relationship effect of perceiver i with target j is

$$\hat{g}_{ij} = X_{ij} - \hat{a}_i - \hat{b}_j - M_{..}$$

The data can be viewed as a two-way design, perceiver × target. For a two-way design, a two-way analysis of variance can be computed. The mean square for perceivers, or MS_P, is defined as

$$\frac{r\Sigma\hat{a}_i^2}{n - 1}$$

The mean square for targets, or MS_t, is defined as

$$\frac{n\Sigma\hat{b}_i^2}{r - 1}$$

The mean square for perceiver × target interaction, or MS_b, is defined as

$$\frac{\Sigma\Sigma\hat{g}_{ij}^2}{(n - 1)(r - 1)}$$

These are the usual two-way analysis of variance mean squares. Because both perceiver and target are random effects, the estimates of the variances are as follows:

$$s_a^2 = \frac{MS_P - MS_I}{r}$$

$$s_b^2 = \frac{MS_T - MS_I}{n}$$

$$s_g^2 = MS_I$$

So this differs from the usual fixed-effects analysis of variance, in that the goal is not to test differences between means, but rather to estimate the variances of the perceiver, target, and relationship effects.

Note that it is possible that both s_a^2 and s_b^2 are estimated as negative. Because negative variances are not interpretable, they are typically set to zero. However, when one is averaging across groups, the negative variance should be retained.

There are simple tests of statistical significance for the perceiver and target variances. They are F tests:

$$F[n-1, (r-1)(n-1)] = \frac{MS_P}{MS_I}$$

$$F[r-1, (r-1)(n-1)] = \frac{MS_T}{MS_I}$$

If the F is significant, then the variance component is needed.

For the example in Table 2.3, $MS_P = 5$, $MS_T = 17.2$, and $MS_I = .95$. The estimates are : $s_a^2 = (5 - .95)/5 = .81$, $s_b^2 = (17.2 - .95)/5 = 3.25$, and $s_g^2 = .95$.

If there are multiple groups of half-blocks, the results can be averaged across groups. Complications in weighting arise if the groups have different numbers of perceivers or targets.

Full-Block Design

In a full-block design, each person serves as both a perceiver and a target, and so there are two half-blocks. There are two subgroups, one with n people and the other with r. The first half-block has n perceivers and r targets. The two people then switch roles, and so there is a second half-block with r perceivers and n targets. One can estimate the variance components for each half-block. That is, one computes mean squares within each and estimates the perceiver, target, and relationship variance. When there is no distinction between the two groups, these two sets of variance components can be averaged. The estimates for perceiver and target variance are weighted by subgroup size minus 1.

With the full-block design, two covariances can be estimated. They are estimated by two mean cross-products: perceiver–target, MCP_{PT}, and inter-action, MCP_I. The formula for MCP_{PT} for the subgroup with n persons is

$$\frac{\Sigma \hat{a}_i \hat{b}_i}{n - 1}$$

where the summation is over n, and for the other subgroup

$$\frac{\Sigma \hat{a}_i \hat{b}_i}{r - 1}$$

where the summation is over r. The single formula for MCP_I is

$$\frac{\Sigma \Sigma \hat{g}_{ij} \hat{g}_{ji}}{(n - 1)(r - 1)}$$

One can then take these mean cross-products and use them to solve for the unknown covariances:

$$s_{ab} = \frac{MCP_{PT} - MCP_I}{n}$$

There is a parallel formula in which the denominator is r. The two estimates of s_{ab} are averaged and weighted by subgroup size minus 1. The relationship covariance is given as:

$$s_{gg'} = MCP_I$$

With these two covariances, it is possible to estimate their parallel correlations. The perceiver–target correlation is estimated by

$$\frac{s_{ab}}{\sqrt{s_a^2 s_b^2}}$$

and the relationship correlation is estimated by

$$\frac{s_{gg'}}{s_g^2}$$

The relationship correlation is bounded by $+1$ and -1. However, as discussed in Chapter 2, the perceiver–target correlation is not bounded by $+1$ and -1. By convention, out-of-range values are set to $+1$ or -1, depending on the sign of the correlation. Many, but not all, out-of-range estimates can be avoided by first determining whether both the perceiver and target variances are significant; if they are not, the correlation is not computed.

The perceiver–target correlation states what the correlation between the perceiver and target effects would be if there were many perceivers and targets. That is, it is a forecast of a correlation if there were virtually an unlimited number of perceivers and targets. Thus, the estimate is not dependent on sample size.

There is no standard significance test available for the block design. The procedure used in SRM analyses is to estimate repeatedly the parameters (σ_a^2, σ_b^2, σ_g^2, σ_{ab}, and $\sigma_{gg'}$) across different groups. Then group is treated as the unit of analysis, and the parameters are averaged across groups. To test whether a variance or a covariance is statistically significant, one performs a one-sample t test in which the degrees of freedom equals the number of groups minus 1. A one-sample t test is simply the mean parameter estimate times the square root of the number of groups, divided by the standard deviation of the parameter estimate across groups. The test's degrees of freedom equals the sample size minus 1. The tests of variance are one-tailed because a variance cannot be negative, and the tests of covariance are two-tailed.

Round-Robin Design

In a round-robin design, all n people rate one another. So there are n perceivers and n targets. For round-robin designs, the estimation procedure is basically the same as it is for the block design: One computes the effect estimates for perceiver, target, and relationship, and with these estimates one computes mean squares and cross-products that can be used to solve for the model's parameters. The formulas are somewhat more complicated, but the procedure is basically the same.

Again, the term $M_{i.}$ symbolizes the mean for perceiver i averaged across $n - 1$ targets; the term $M_{.j}$ symbolizes the mean for target j averaged across $n - 1$ perceivers; and the term $M_{..}$ symbolizes the mean across all $n(n - 1)$ observations.

The estimate of the perceiver effect for perceiver i is

$$\hat{a}_i = \frac{(n - 1)^2}{n(n - 2)} M_{i.} + \frac{n - 1}{n(n - 2)} M_{.i} - \frac{n - 1}{n - 2} M_{..}$$

The estimate of the target effect for target i is

$$\hat{b}_i = \frac{(n - 1)^2}{n(n - 2)} M_{.i} + \frac{n - 1}{n(n - 2)} M_{i.} - \frac{n - 1}{n - 2} M_{..}$$

The estimate of the relationship effect for perceiver i's rating of target j is

$$\hat{g}_{ij} = X_{ij} - \hat{a}_i - \hat{b}_j - M_{..}$$

The following mean squares are estimated:

$$A = \frac{\Sigma \hat{a}_i^2}{n - 1}$$

$$B = \frac{\Sigma \hat{b}_i^2}{n - 1}$$

$$C = \frac{\Sigma \hat{a}_i \hat{b}_i}{n - 1}$$

The summation is across n persons.

For the relationship effects, the average and the difference are defined:

$$\hat{e}_{ij} = .5(\hat{g}_{ij} + \hat{g}_{ji})$$
$$\hat{d}_{ij} = \hat{g}_{ij} - \hat{g}_{ji}$$

Then, summing across the $n(n - 1)/2$ dyads, the following mean squares are computed:

$$D = \frac{2\Sigma \hat{e}_{ij}^2}{[(n - 1)(n - 2)/2] - 1}$$

$$E = \frac{\Sigma \hat{d}_{ij}^2}{(n - 1)(n - 2)}$$

The estimate of the relationship variance, or s_g^2, equals

$$\frac{D + E}{2}$$

The estimate of the relationship covariance, or $s_{gg'}$, equals

$$\frac{D - E}{2}$$

The estimate of actor–partner covariance equals

$$C - \frac{s_{gg'}(n - 1)}{n(n - 2)} - \frac{s_g^2}{n(n - 2)}$$

The estimate of the perceiver variance equals

$$A - \frac{s_g^2 (n - 1)}{n(n - 2)} - \frac{s_{gg'}}{n(n - 2)}$$

The estimate of the target variance equals

$$B - \frac{s_g^2 (n - 1)}{n(n - 2)} - \frac{s_{gg'}}{n(n - 2)}$$

Significance testing for the round-robin design proceeds as with the block design. The estimate is computed for each group, and it is tested by a one-sample t test to determine whether the mean of the estimates is significantly different from 0. If group sizes vary, estimates are weighted by $n - 1$. That is, the mean and the variance are weighted estimates.

Bivariate Relationships

So far, the discussion has been limited to a single variable. Considered now is the correlation between two variables, X and Y. Surprisingly, with two variables there are six possible correlations—four at the individual level and two at the dyadic level. The four correlations at the individual level are perceiver–perceiver, perceiver–target, target–perceiver, and target–target, where the first term stands for X and the second for Y.

At the dyadic level, there is both an intrapersonal and an interpersonal correlation. The intrapersonal correlation is between the two variables with the same perceiver and target; the interpersonal correlation refers to the case in which the perceiver and target are reversed. So, for example, for the variables of liking and intelligence, the intrapersonal correlation measures the correlation between how much a perceiver especially likes a target and how much the perceiver particularly sees the target as intelligent. The interpersonal correlation measures the correlation between how much a perceiver especially likes a target and how much that target particularly sees the perceiver as intelligent.

Estimation and Testing

The measurement of bivariate correlations is considered for the round-robin design. (The formulas for the half-block and full-block designs can be easily generalized from the univariate formulas.) The SRM formula for the second variable, Y, is as follows:

$$Y_{ij} = p + c_i + f_j + h_{ij}$$

where p is the constant, c_i the perceiver effect, d_j the target effect, and h_{ij} the relationship effect for variable Y. The effect estimates for Y are computed as they are for X. The following covariances are computed:

$$A = \frac{\Sigma \hat{a}_i \hat{c}_i}{n - 1}$$

$$B = \frac{\Sigma \hat{a}_i \hat{f}_i}{n - 1}$$

$$C = \frac{\Sigma \hat{b}_i \hat{c}_i}{n - 1}$$

$$D = \frac{\Sigma \hat{b}_i \hat{f}_i}{n - 1}$$

The following terms, analogous to d_{ij} and e_{ij}, are defined:

$$\hat{t}_{ij} = .5(\hat{h}_{ij} + \hat{h}_{ji})$$
$$\hat{s}_{ij} = \hat{h}_{ij} - \hat{h}_{ji}$$

Then, summing across the $n(n - 1)/2$ dyads, the following two mean cross-products are computed:

$$E = \frac{2\Sigma \hat{c}_{ij} \hat{t}_{ij}}{[(n - 1)(n - 2)/2] - 1}$$

$$F = \frac{\Sigma \hat{d}_{ij} \hat{s}_{ij}}{(n - 1)(n - 2)}$$

The intrapersonal relationship covariance, or s_{gh}, is estimated by

$$\frac{E + F}{2}$$

The interpersonal relationship covariance, or $s_{gh'}$, is estimated by

$$\frac{E - F}{2}$$

The perceiver–perceiver covariance is estimated by

$$A - \frac{s_{gh}(n-1)}{n(n-2)} - \frac{s_{gh'}}{n(n-2)}$$

The perceiver–target covariance is estimated by

$$B - \frac{s_{gh'}(n-1)}{n(n-2)} - \frac{s_{gh}}{n(n-2)}$$

The target–perceiver covariance is estimated by

$$C - \frac{s_{gh'}(n-1)}{n(n-2)} - \frac{s_{gh}}{n(n-2)}$$

The target–target covariance is estimated by

$$D - \frac{s_{gh}(n-1)}{n(n-2)} - \frac{s_{gh'}}{n(n-2)}$$

The previously presented univariate estimates can be shown to be a special case of the bivariate estimates (i.e., when $X_{ij} = Y_{ij}$).

To compute correlations, each of these covariances is divided by the square root of the product of the variances of the terms that make up the covariance. So the perceiver–target covariance is divided by the square root of the product of the perceiver variance for X and the target variance for Y. Like the univariate perceiver–target correlations, these correlations can be out of range.

The unit of analysis in significance tests is the group. The estimate is computed for each group, and a one-sample t test is used to test the mean against the null hypothesis that it is 0. The mean of the estimates is tested to determine whether it is significantly different from 0. Tests of covariance are two-tailed.

Personality Measures and Self-Measures

Sometimes the variable Y contains only perceiver variance. For instance, if Y is a measure of the age or the intelligence of the perceiver, then Y will not have target or relationship variance. For such a variable, only the perceiver–perceiver and target–perceiver covariances are defined. Because there is no relationship variance, the two relationship covariances are not defined.

A self-measure has only perceiver variance. A person's self-rating does not ordinarily vary across targets. If it does vary (e.g., a person rates himself or herself after each interaction), all four covariances can be computed.

For a self-measure and a personality measure, standard tests of significance of the covariances are possible. First, the perceiver and target effects are computed for X. Then an ordinary Pearson product–moment correlation can be computed between these estimates and Y, partialing out groups. Basically, correlations are computed within each group and pooled. This correlation can be tested for statistical significance in the usual way, with degrees of freedom of $N - G - 1$, where N is the number of people and G the number of groups.

It is possible to regress self-measures on perceiver and target effects. The unstandardized regression coefficient for perceiver is the term called k in Chapter 9, and the coefficient for target is the term called q. The unexplained variance in the regression equation can be considered self–relationship variance.

Construct Effects

To separate error from relationship variance, there must be multiple replications or measures of the theoretical construct. Replications are obtained by measuring the construct at more than one time or by multiple indicators. If there are replications, all four terms in the model—mean, perceiver, target, and relationship—can be partitioned into stable and unstable components. Generally, there is not much interest in the partitioning of the mean, but there is interest in the other three sources.

Formally, SRM with multiple measures is as follows:

$$X_{ijk} = m + m_k + a_i + a_{ik} + b_j + b_{jk} + g_{ij} + g_{ijk}$$

where subscript k refers to measure. The seven terms with subscripts are all random variables with zero mean. They are defined as follows:

Mean unstable, or m_k: Mean differences between measures.
Perceiver stable, or a_i: Perceiver variance that replicates across measures.
Perceiver unstable, or a_{ik}: Perceiver variance that is unique to each measure.
Target stable, or b_j: Target variance that replicates across measures.
Target unstable, or b_{jk}: Target variance that is unique to each measure.
Relationship stable, or g_{ij}: Relationship variance that replicates across measures.
Relationship unstable, or g_{ijk}: Relationship variance that is unique to each measure.

If the measures are carefully chosen, there is usually little unstable perceiver and target variance, and so the only unstable variance is relationship variance, which is treated as error. If the unstable mean, perceiver, and target terms are dropped, the model is SRM as originally presented (Warner, Kenny, & Stoto, 1979):

$$X_{ijk} = m + a_i + b_j + g_{ij} + g_{ijk}$$

The Warner et al. (1979) assumptions generally hold in that often there is little or no unstable perceiver or target variance. However, it is usually not the case that the means of the indicators are identical, and so the Warner et al. (1979) assumption of no m_k term is likely to be false.

In presentations of construct variance partitioning, the unstable mean variance is usually ignored. The proportion of stable perceiver, target, and relationship variance is presented, and the unstable sources are lumped together as error. In certain applications, it is useful to present all seven sources of variance (Hallmark & Kenny, 1989). For instance, in Chapter 3 the unstable perceiver variance has been used.

There are two ways to approach the estimation of construct variances: first, by using mean squares from analysis of variance; second, through the pooling of covariances. Both of these approaches are described.

Mean Squares

Consider the case of the half-block design, in which n perceivers judge r targets on q measures. I denote the measures factor as R. The data structure is a three-way design. There are seven sources of variance: MS_P, MS_T, MS_R, $MS_{P \times T}$, $MS_{P \times R}$, $MS_{T \times R}$, and $MS_{P \times T \times R}$. It is assumed that all three factors are random. Formulas for estimating the seven sources of variance are presented in most advanced textbooks on analysis of variance, and they are represented here.

The estimate of stable perceiver variance is as follows:

$$\frac{MS_P - MS_{P \times T} - MS_{P \times R} + MS_{P \times T \times R}}{rq}$$

Stable target variance:

$$\frac{MS_T - MS_{P \times T} - MS_{T \times R} + MS_{P \times T \times R}}{nq}$$

Stable relationship variance:

$$\frac{MS_{P \times T} - MS_{P \times T \times R}}{q}$$

Unstable perceiver variance:

$$\frac{MS_{P \times R} - MS_{P \times T \times R}}{r}$$

Unstable target variance:

$$\frac{MS_{T \times R} - MS_{P \times T \times R}}{n}$$

Finally, the estimate of unstable relationship variance is $MS_{P \times T \times R}$.

Formulas for the full-block design are rather straightforward; analyses of variance are done within each block and then pooled. However, for the round-robin design the estimation procedure is quite complicated, and a second approach is to be preferred.

Average of Covariance Matrices

The second approach uses the variances and covariances between measures to estimate the construct variances and covariances. Consider the simple example in which there are three indicators — 1, 2, and 3 — of a construct. Each covariance matrix of the three measures (e.g., perceiver–perceiver) can be represented as follows:

	1	2	3
1	$C(1,1)$	$C(1,2)$	$C(1,3)$
2	$C(2,1)$	$C(2,2)$	$C(2,3)$
3	$C(3,1)$	$C(3,2)$	$C(3,3)$

This is a symmetric matrix, and so $C(1,2)$ equals $C(2,1)$.

The stable perceiver variance is given by the average of the off-diagonal elements, or

$$\frac{C(1,2) + C(1,3) + C(2,3)}{3}$$

The unstable perceiver variance is given by the average of the diagonal minus the average of the off-diagonal elements, or

$$\frac{C(1,1) + C(2,2) + C(3,3)}{3} - \frac{C(1,2) + C(1,3) + C(2,3)}{3}$$

Surprisingly, this value gives the same answer as the previously described mean-square method. However, it is much simpler to compute and can be used with any design.

Estimates of the other variances and covariances (e.g., perceiver–target) can be obtained in a similar fashion. The stable variance equals the average of the off-diagonal estimates, and the unstable variance equals the average of the diagonal elements minus the stable variance.

For those familiar with measurement models in structural equation modeling (e.g., LISREL), it is useful to describe the measurement model within that approach. Each variable is assumed to load on a common factor, and all of the loadings are fixed to 1. In essence, the loadings are all set equal to one another.

Conclusion

The formulas for the estimates of SRM parameters can be fairly complicated, but they are straightforward. Unfortunately, standard computer packages (e.g., SAS and SPSS) cannot be easily used. All of the computations described in this appendix have been computer-programmed. The computer program SOREMO (Kenny, 1993a) was developed for the analysis of round-robin designs, and BLOCKO (Kenny, 1993b) was developed for block designs. Both programs are written in FORTRAN for IBM-compatible personal computers.

Another major limitation of this approach is that one of the designs must be used and there must be no missing data. Work is currently underway to relax these requirements.

THE WEIGHTED-AVERAGE MODEL OF PERCEPTION

The model discussed in this appendix is an elaboration of a model first presented elsewhere (Kenny, 1991), called the Weighted-Average Model (WAM). This appendix presents a more general version of WAM plus proofs of various formulas. Because of the proofs and the number of terms in the model, the content of this appendix is much more complex than the material in the chapters. The reader may wish to review the section in Chapter 4 on WAM before reading this appendix. Table C.1 presents the 11 model parameters.

TABLE C.1. Parameters of WAM

Parameter	Definition
n	Acquaintance (number of acts)
q	Overlap
r_1	Within-judge consistency
r_2	Similar meaning systems
r_3	Between-judge consistency
w	Weight of physical-appearance stereotypes
r_4	Agreement about stereotypes
r_5	Assumed "kernel of truth" in stereotypes (within a judge)
r_6	"Kernel of truth" (between judges)
k	Weight of unique impression (extraneous information)
a	Communication

Note. In Kenny (1991), w was set to 0, and it was assumed that $r_3 = r_1r_2$. In Chapter 4 of this text, to simplify discussion, it has been assumed that $r_3 = r_1r_2$, and that $r_6 = r_4r_5$. Also, r_4 here is denoted in Chapter 4 as r_3, and r_5 here is denoted there as r_4.

Parts of this appendix are adapted from Kenny, Albright, Malloy, and Kashy (in press). Copyright 1994 by the American Psychological Association. Adapted by permission.

Model Parameters

Consider a target who engages in a series of acts. Perceivers 1 and 2 each see n of the acts. A total of qn acts is seen in common, where q is less than or equal to 1. The parameter q is referred to as the overlap parameter. A perceiver's impression of a target depends on three sources of information: the n acts, the perceiver's unique impression, and physical-appearance information. Attached to each is a scale value or the meaning that the perceiver gives to the information. The scale values for the act are denoted as s_1, s_2, and so on. The unique impression's scale value is denoted as s_0, and the scale value for physical appearance is s_P. Each of these scale values is double-subscripted below; the first subscript denotes the perceiver and the second the act.

The formulas for the impressions of perceiver 1 (I_1) and perceiver 2 (I_2) are as follows:

$$I_1 = \frac{w s_{1P} + \Sigma s_{1i} + k s_{10}}{n + w + k}$$

$$I_2 = \frac{w s_{2P} + \Sigma s_{2i} + k s_{20}}{n + w + k}$$

The term w is the weight of physical-appearance stereotypes, and k is the weight of the unique impression; k and w are assumed to be the same for both perceivers.

The denominator can be ignored because correlations are not affected by a constant. So the $n + w + k$ term can be ignored. The variances of all terms equal o_s^2 where the variances are computed across targets within a judge. If the variances do differ, that difference can be expressed in terms of the weights. All expected values are zero except the unique impression.

The correlations between scale values are as follows:

	s_{11}	s_{12}	s_{21}	s_{22}	s_{1P}	s_{2P}
s_{11}	1					
s_{12}	r_1	1				
s_{21}	r_2	r_3	1			
s_{22}	r_3	r_2	r_1	1		
s_{1P}	r_5	r_5	r_6	r_6	1	
s_{2P}	r_6	r_6	r_5	r_5	r_4	1

All the correlations between the scale values of the unique impressions, s_{10} and s_{20}, are all zero. The definitions of the six correlations are as follows:

r_1: Consistency within a judge across acts.
r_2: Agreement between judges within an act.
r_3: Consistency between judges across acts.
r_4: Agreement between judges on physical-appearance stereotypes.
r_5: Assumed consistency within a judge between physical-appearance stereotypes and an act.
r_6: Consistency between a judge's evaluation of physical appearance and another judge's evaluation of an act.

The last parameter can be viewed as a "kernel of truth" parameter, because it represents the correlation between the "truth" (the target's behavior) and the stereotype that the perceiver has concerning the target's behavior. The correlation between s_{1P} and I_1 where n is very large is $r_5/\sqrt{r_1}$, and the correlation between s_{1P} and I_2 where n is very large is $r_6/\sqrt{r_3}$.

The six correlations are not independent. So, for instance, if both r_1 and r_2 are assumed to equal 1, it must be the case that r_3 also equals 1. Earlier (Kenny, 1991), I assumed that $r_3 = r_1 r_2$. In Chapter 4, it has been assumed that $r_6 = r_4 r_5$ and that $r_3 = r_1 r_2$ (all terms as defined here). Also, to simplify the presentation of the model in the text, what is called r_4 here is called r_3 in the text, and what is called r_5 here is called r_4 in the text.

Consensus (c)

To determine consensus (c), or the correlation between I_1 and I_2, first the variance of I_1 and I_2 is determined, and then the covariance between I_1 and I_2 is determined. The variance, or o_I^2, equals

$$o_I^2 = o_s^2[k^2 + w^2 + n + n(n-1)r_1 + 2wr_s]$$
$$= o_s^2[k^2 + w^2 + n(1 + (n-1)r_1) + 2wr_s]$$

The covariance between I_1 and I_2 does not involve the s_0 terms because they are independent. A total of qn of the s terms are the same, and $(1 - q)n$ are different. There are then five components of covariance: the covariance between the overlapping terms (A), the covariance between the nonoverlapping terms (B), the covariance between the two (C), the agreement between s_{1P} and s_{2P} (D), and the covariance between the scale values of the physical appearance and the behaviors (E). They are as follows:

$$A = qno_s^2 r_2 + qn(qn-1)o_s^2 r_3$$
$$B = (1-q)^2 n^2 o_s^2 r_3$$
$$C = 2q(1-q)n^2 o_s^2 r_3$$
$$D = w^2 o_s^2 r_4$$
$$E = 2wno_s^2 r_6$$

Notice that in A, B, and C, there are a number of terms containing $\sigma_s^2 r_3$. The sum of those terms is

$$qn(qn - 1) + (1 - q)^2 n^2 + 2q(1 - q)n^2$$

which equals

$$q^2 n^2 - qn + n^2 - 2qn^2 + q^2 n^2 + 2qn^2 - 2q^2 n^2$$

This simplifies to $n^2 - qn$. So the covariance between I_1 and I_2 equals

$$\sigma_s^2 [w^2 r_4 + 2wnr_6 + qnr_2 + (n^2 - qn)r_3]$$

The value of c equals the covariance between I_1 and I_2 divided by the variance of I. Note that the σ_s^2 terms cancel to produce the following:

$$c = \frac{w^2 r_4 + 2wnr_6 + qnr_2 + (n^2 - qn)r_3}{k^2 + w^2 + n[1 + r_1(n - 1) + 2wr_5]}$$

Note that when $w = r_4 = r_5 = 0$ and $r_3 = r_1 r_2$, the formula above reduces to formula 2 in Kenny (1991). Note that as n increases, c approaches r_3/r_1, which in the simpler version of the model equals r_2.

To allow for communication effects, the impression for judge 1 is

$$I_1' = aI_2 + I_1$$

The variance of I_1' is

$$V(aI_2 + I_1) = \sigma_I^2(a^2 + 1 + 2ac)$$

and the covariance between the two impressions is

$$C(aI_1 + I_2, aI_2 + I_1) = \sigma_I^2(a^2 c + 2a + c)$$

Therefore c', the consensus correlation allowing for communication, equals

$$\frac{\sigma_I^2(a^2 c + 2a + c)}{\sigma_I^2(a^2 c + 1 + 2ac)}$$

which reduces to

$$\frac{c + a^2 c + 2a}{1 + a^2 + 2ac}$$

This formula is identical to formula 3 in Kenny (1991).

Accuracy (v)

The accuracy correlation is symbolized by v, which stands for validity. The criterion score is assumed to be $\Sigma I_i/p$, or the average of all possible impressions, where p symbolizes the number of possible impressions. The correlation between I_1 and $\Sigma I_i/p$ is now determined. First, the variance of I_1 is defined as

$$\frac{\sigma_s^2[k^2 + w^2 + n(1 + r_1(n - 1)) + 2wr_5]}{(n + k + w)^2}$$

The variance of $\Sigma I_i/p$ is $\sigma_s^2 r_3$. The covariance between I_1 and $\Sigma I_i/p$ is

$$\frac{\sigma_s^2(wr_6 + nr_3)}{n + k + w}$$

The validity correlation, or v, equals

$$\frac{wr_6 + nr_3)}{\sqrt{r_3(k^2 + w^2 + n[1 + r_1(n - 1)] + 2wr_5)}}$$

If there is communication, then the correlation equals

$$\frac{v(1 + a)}{\sqrt{1 + a^2 + 2ac}}$$

REFERENCES

Abelson, R. P., & Miller, J. (1967). Negative persuasion via personal insult. *Journal of Experimental Social Psychology, 3*, 321–333.

Albright, I. (1990). [A longitudinal study of consensus and accuracy in interpersonal perception.] Unpublished raw data, Westfield State College.

Albright, L., Kenny, D. A., & Malloy, T. E. (1988). Consensus in personality judgments at zero acquaintance. *Journal of Personality and Social Psychology, 55*, 387–395.

Albright, L., Malloy, T. E., Kenny, D. A., & Borkenau, P. (1994). *Validity in personality judgments at zero acquaintance.* Unpublished manuscript, Westfield State College.

Albright-Malloy, L. (1988). The role of acquaintance in accuracy of interpersonal perception (Doctoral dissertation, University of Connecticut, 1987). *Dissertation Abstracts International, 48*, 3448A.

Alloy, L. B., & Abramson, L. Y. (1988). Depressive realism: Four theoretical perspectives. In L. B. Alloy (Ed.), *Cognitive processes in depression* (pp. 223–265). New York: Guilford Press.

Ambady, N., & Rosenthal, R. (1992). Thin slices of expressive behavior as predictors of interpersonal consequences: A meta-analysis. *Psychological Bulletin, 111*, 256–274.

Anderson, N. (1981). *Foundations of information integration theory.* New York: Academic Press.

Anderson, R. (1985). Measuring social self-perception: How accurately can individuals predict how others view them? (Doctoral dissertation, University of Connecticut, 1984). *Dissertation Abstracts International, 45*, 3610A.

Aron, A., & Aron, E. N. (1986). *Love and the expansion of self: Understanding attraction and satisfaction.* Washington, DC: Hemisphere.

Asch, S. E. (1946). Forming impressions of personality. *Journal of Abnormal and Social Psychology, 41*(3), 258–290.

Ausubel, D. P., & Schiff, H. M., & Gasser, E. B. (1952). A preliminary study of developmental trends in socioempathy: Accuracy of perception of own and others' sociometric status. *Child Development, 23*, 111–128.

Barefoot, J. C. (1991). Developments in the measurement of hostility. In H. Friedman (Ed.), *Hostility, coping, and health* (pp. 13–31). Washington, DC: American Psychological Association.

Baron, R. M., & Misovich, S. J. (1993). Dispositional knowing from an ecological perspective. *Personality and Social Psychology Bulletin, 19,* 541–552.

Baumeister, R. F. (1982). A self-presentational view of social phenomena. *Psychological Bulletin, 91,* 3–26.

Beck, A. T. (1967). *Depression: Clinical, experimental, and theoretical aspects.* New York: Harper & Row.

Bem, D. J. (1967). Self perception: An alternative interpretation of cognitive dissonance phenomena. *Psychological Review, 74,* 183–200.

Berglas, S., & Jones, E. E. (1978). Drug choice as an externalization strategy in response to noncontingent success. *Journal of Personality and Social Psychology, 36,* 405–417.

Bernard, H. R., Killworth, P. D., & Sailer, L. (1982). Informant accuracy in social network data V: An experimental attempt to predict actual communication from recall data. *Social Science Research, 11,* 30–66.

Berry, D. S. (1990). Taking people at face value: Evidence for the kernel of truth hypothesis. *Social Cognition, 8,* 343–361.

Berscheid, E., & Walster, E. H. (1978). *Interpersonal attraction* (2nd ed.). Reading, MA: Addison-Wesley.

Blumberg, H. H. (1972). Communication of interpersonal evaluations. *Journal of Personality and Social Psychology, 23,* 157–162.

Bohrnstedt, G. W., & Felson, R. B. (1983). Explaining the relations among children's actual and perceived performances and self-esteem: A comparison of several causal models. *Journal of Personality and Social Psychology, 45,* 43–56.

Bond, C. F., Jr., Kahler, K. N., & Paolicelli, L. M. (1985). The miscommunication of deception: An adaptive perspective. *Journal of Experimental Social Psychology, 21,* 331–345.

Borkenau, P. (1990). Traits as ideal-based and goal-derived social categories. *Journal of Personality and Social Psychology, 58,* 381–396.

Borkenau, P., & Liebler, A. (1992). Trait inferences: Sources of validity at zero acquaintance. *Journal of Personality and Social Psychology, 62,* 645–657.

Bourne, E. (1977). Can we describe an individual's personality? Agreement on stereotype versus individual attributes. *Journal of Personality and Social Psychology, 35,* 863–872.

Bronfenbrenner, U., Harding, J., & Gallwey, M. (1958). The measurement of skill in social perception. In D. C. McClelland, A. L. Baldwin, U. Bronfenbrenner, & F. L. Strodtbeck (Eds.), *Talent and society* (pp. 29–111). Princeton, NJ: Van Nostrand.

Brunswik, E. (1956). *Perception and the representative design of psychological experiments* (2nd ed.). Berkeley, CA: University of California Press.

Buck, R. (1984). *The communication of emotion.* New York: Guilford Press.

Burger, J. M. (1981). Motivational biases in the attribution of responsibility for an accident: A meta-analysis of the defensive attribution hypothesis. *Psychological Bulletin, 90,* 496–512.

Burleson, J. A. (1983). Reciprocity of interpersonal attraction within acquainted versus unacquainted small groups (Doctoral dissertation, University of Texas, 1982). *Dissertation Abstracts International, 43,* 4194A.

Byrne, D. (1971). *The attraction paradigm.* New York: Academic Press.

Campbell, D. T. (1961). Conformity in psychology's theories of acquired behavioral dispositions. In I. A. Berg & B. M. Bass (Eds.), *Conformity and deviation* (pp. 101–142). New York: Harper & Row.

Campbell, D. T. (1979). A tribal model of the social system vehicle carrying scientific knowledge. *Knowledge, 2,* 181–201.

Campbell, D. T., & Fiske, D. W. (1959). Convergent and discriminant validation by the multitrait–multimethod matrix. *Psychological Bulletin, 56,* 81–105.

Campbell, D. T., Miller, N., Lubetsky, J., & O'Connell, E. J. (1964). Varieties of projection in trait attribution. *Psychological Monographs, 78* (Whole No. 592).

Campbell, J. D., & Fehr, B. (1990). Self-esteem and perceptions of conveyed impressions: Is negative affectivity associated with greater realism? *Journal of Personality and Social Psychology, 58,* 122–133.

Cappella, J. C. (1981). Mutual influence in expressive behavior: Adult–adult and infant–adult dyadic interaction. *Psychological Bulletin, 89,* 101–132.

Chapdelaine, A., Kenny, D. A., & LaFontana, K. M. (in press). Matchmaker, matchmaker, can you make me a match?: Predicting liking between two unacquainted persons. *Journal of Personality and Social Psychology.*

Cline, V. B. (1964). Interpersonal perception. In B. Maher (Ed.), *Progress in experimental personality research* (Vol. 1, pp. 221–284). New York: Academic Press.

Cline, V. B., & Richards, J. M., Jr. (1960). Accuracy of interpersonal perception: A general trait? *Journal of Abnormal and Social Psychology, 60,* 1–7.

Cook, M. (1979). *Perceiving others: The psychology of interpersonal perception.* London: Methuen.

Cooley, C. H. (1902). *Human nature and the social order* (rev. ed.) New York: Scribner's.

Costa, P. T., Jr., & McCrae, R. R. (1985). *The NEO Personality Inventory manual.* Odessa, FL: Psychological Assessment Resources.

Cronbach, L. J. (1955). Processes affecting scores on "understanding of others" and "assumed similarity." *Psychological Bulletin, 52,* 177–193.

Cronbach, L. J. (1958). Proposals leading to analytic treatment of social perception scores. In R. Tagiuri & L. Petrullo (Eds.), *Person perception and interpersonal behavior* (pp. 353–379). Stanford, CA: Stanford University Press.

Cronbach, L. J., Gleser, G. C., Nanda, H., & Rajaratnam, N. (1972). *The dependability of behavioral measurements: Theory of generalizability for scores and profiles.* New York: Wiley.

Crow, W. J., & Hammond, K. R. (1957). The generality of accuracy and response sets in interpersonal perception. *Journal of Abnormal and Social Psychology, 54,* 384–390.

Crowne, D. P., & Marlowe, D. (1960). A new scale of social desirability independent of psychopathology. *Journal of Consulting Psychology, 24,* 349–354.

Crozier, W. R. (1979). Shyness as a dimension of personality. *British Journal of Social and Clinical Psychology, 18,* 121–128.

Curry, T. J., & Emerson, R. M. (1970). Balance theory: A theory of interpersonal attraction? *Sociometry, 33,* 216–238.

Dabbs, J. M., Jr., & Ruback, R. B. (1987). Dimensions of group process: Amount and structure of vocal interaction. In L. Berkowitz (Ed.), *Advances in experimental social psychology*, (Vol. 20, pp. 123–169). San Diego, CA: Academic Press.

Dantchik, A. (1985). *Idiographic approaches to personality assessment*. Unpublished manuscript, Arizona State University.

DePaulo, B. M. (1992). Nonverbal behavior and self-presentation. *Psychological Bulletin, 111*, 203–243.

DePaulo, B. M., Kenny, D. A., Hoover, C., Webb, W., & Oliver, P. V. (1987). Accuracy of person perception: Do people know what kind of impressions they convey? *Journal of Personality and Social Psychology, 52*, 303–315.

DePaulo, B. M., & Rosenthal, R. (1982). Measuring the development of sensitivity to nonverbal communication. In C. E. Izard (Ed.), *Measuring emotions in infants and children* (pp. 208–247). New York: Cambridge University Press.

DePaulo, B. M., Rosenthal, R., Eisenstat, R. A., Rogers, P. L., & Finkelstein, S. (1978). Decoding discrepant nonverbal cues. *Journal of Personality and Social Psychology, 36*, 313–323.

DePaulo, B. M., Stone, J. I., & Lassiter, G. D. (1985). Deceiving and detecting deceit. In B. R. Schlenker (Ed.), *The self and social life* (pp. 323–370). New York: McGraw-Hill.

DiPilato, M. (1990). Person perception in initial acquaintanceship: Changes over time and task–trait match (Doctoral dissertation, Arizona State University, 1989). *Dissertation Abstracts International, 51*, 1038A.

Dodge, K. A., & Coie, J. D. (1987). Social-information-processing factors in reactive and proactive aggression in children's peer groups. *Journal of Personality and Social Psychology, 53*, 1146–1158.

Dornbusch, S. M., Hastorf, A. H., Richardson, S. A., Muzzy, R. E., & Vreeland, R. S. (1965). The perceiver and the perceived: Their relative influence on categories of interpersonal cognition. *Journal of Personality and Social Psychology, 1*, 434–440.

Felson, R. B. (1980). Communication barriers and the reflected appraisal process. *Social Psychology Quarterly, 43*, 223–233.

Felson, R. B. (1981). Self- and reflected appraisal among football players: A test of the Meadian hypothesis. *Social Psychology Quarterly, 44*, 116–126.

Felson, R. B. (1989). Parents and reflected appraisal process: A longitudinal analysis. *Journal of Personality and Social Psychology, 56*, 965–971.

Felson, R. B. (1992). Coming to see ourselves: Social sources of self appraisal. *Advances in Group Processes, 9*, 185–205.

Fenigstein, A., Scheier, M. F., & Buss, A. H. (1975). Public and private self-consciousness: Assessment and theory. *Journal of Consulting and Clinical Psychology, 43*, 522–527.

Fishbein, M., & Ajzen, I. (1975). *Belief, attitude, intention, and behavior: An introduction to theory and research*. Reading, MA: Addison-Wesley.

Fiske, S. T. (1993). Social cognition and social perception. *Annual Review of Psychology, 44*, 155–194.

Fiske, S. T., & Cox, M. (1979). Person concepts: The effect of target familiarity and descriptive purpose on the process of describing others. *Journal of Personality, 47*, 136–161.

Flink, C., & Park, B. (1991). Increasing consensus in trait judgments through outcome dependency. *Journal of Experimental Social Psychology, 27,* 453–467.

Folkes, V. S., & Sears, D. O. (1977). Does everybody like a liker? *Journal of Experimental Social Psychology, 13,* 505–519.

Forgas, J. P. (1992). Affect and social perception: Research evidence and an integrative theory. In W. Stroebe & M. Hewstone (Eds.), *European review of social psychology* (Vol. 3, pp. 183–223). Chichester, England: Wiley.

Frey, K. P., & Smith, E. R. (1993). Beyond the actor's traits: Forming impressions of actors, targets, and relationships from social behaviors. *Journal of Personality and Social Psychology, 65,* 486–493.

Funder, D. C. (1980). On seeing ourselves as others see us: Self–other agreement and discrepancy in personality ratings. *Journal of Personality, 48,* 473–493.

Funder, D. C. (1987). Errors and mistakes: Evaluating the accuracy of social judgment. *Psychological Bulletin, 101,* 75–90.

Funder, D. C., & Colvin, C. R. (1988). Friends and strangers: Acquaintanceship, agreement, and the accuracy of personality judgment. *Journal of Personality and Social Psychology, 55,* 149–158.

Funder, D. C., & Dobroth, K. M. (1987). Differences between traits: Properties associated with interjudge agreement. *Journal of Personality and Social Psychology, 52,* 409–418.

Gage, N. L., & Cronbach, L. J. (1955). Conceptual and methodological problems in interpersonal perception. *Psychological Review, 62,* 411–422.

Gage, N. L., Leavitt, G. S., & Stone, G. C. (1956). The intermediary key in the analysis of interpersonal perception. *Psychological Bulletin, 53,* 258–266.

Gidron, D., Koehler, D. J., & Tversky, A. (1993). Implicit quantification of personality traits. *Personality and Social Psychology Bulletin, 19,* 594–604.

Gilbert, D. T. (1991). How mental systems believe. *American Psychologist, 46,* 107–119.

Gilbert, D. T., & Jones, E. E. (1986). Perceiver-induced constraint: Interpretations of self-generated reality. *Journal of Personality and Social Psychology, 50,* 269–280.

Goffman, E. (1959). *The presentation of self in everyday life.* Garden City, NY: Doubleday.

Goldberg, L. R. (1990). An alternative "description of personality": The Big-Five factor structure. *Journal of Personality and Social Psychology, 59,* 1216–1229.

Gouldner, A. W. (1960). The norm of reciprocity: A preliminary statement. *American Sociological Review, 25,* 161–178.

Guilford, J. P. (1954). *Psychometric methods.* New York: McGraw-Hill.

Hallmark, B. W. (1991). *Leadership, friendliness, and productivity in problem solving small groups.* Unpublished master's thesis, University of Connecticut.

Hallmark, B. W., & Kenny, D. A. (1989). *The effect of rating a person at a time or a trait at a time on the variance components of the Social Relations Model.* Unpublished manuscript, University of Connecticut.

Harackiewicz, J. M., & DePaulo, B. M. (1982). Accuracy of person perception: A component analysis according to Cronbach. *Personality and Social Psychology Bulletin, 8,* 247–256.

Hastie, R., & Rasinski, K. A. (1988). The concept of accuracy in social judgment. In D. Bar-Tal & A. W. Kruglanski (Eds.), *The social psychology of knowledge* (pp. 193–208). Cambridge, England: Cambridge University Press.

Hazan, C., & Shaver, P. R. (1987). Romantic love conceptualized as an attachment process. *Journal of Personality and Social Psychology, 52,* 511–524.

Higgins, E. T., & Bargh, J. A. (1987). Social cognition and social perception. *Annual Review of Psychology, 38,* 369–425.

Higgins, E. T., Herman, C. P., & Zanna, M. P. (Eds.). (1981). *Social cognition: The Ontario Symposium* (Vol. 1). Hillsdale, NJ: Erlbaum.

Ingraham, L. J., & Wright, T. L. (1986). A cautionary note on the interpretation of relationship effects in the Social Relations Model. *Social Psychology Quarterly, 49,* 93–97.

Jackson, D. N. (1972). A model for inferential accuracy. *Canadian Psychologist, 13,* 185–195.

John, O. P., & Robins, R. W. (1993). Determinants of interjudge agreement on personality traits: The big five domains, observability, evaluativeness, and the unique perspective of the self. *Journal of Personality, 61,* 521–551.

John, O. P., & Robins, R. W. (1994). Accuracy and bias in self-perception: Individual differences in self-enhancement and the role of narcissism. *Journal of Personality and Social Psychology, 66,* 206–219.

Jones, E. E. (1964). *Ingratiation: A social psychological analysis.* New York: Appleton-Century-Crofts.

Jones, E. E. (1985). Major developments in social psychology during the past five decades. In G. Lindzey & E. Aronson (Eds.), *The handbook of social psychology* (3rd ed., Vol. 1, pp. 47–107). New York: Random House.

Jones, E. E. (1990). *Interpersonal perception.* New York: Freeman.

Jones, E. E., & Nisbett, R. E. (1971). The actor and the observer: Divergent perceptions of the causes of behavior. In E. E. Jones, D. E. Kanouse, H. H. Kelley, R. E. Nisbett, S. Valins, & B. Weiner (Eds.), *Attribution: Perceiving the causes of behavior* (pp. 79–94). Morristown, NJ: General Learning Press.

Jones, L. E. (1983). Multidimensional models of social perception, cognition, and behavior. *Applied Psychological Measurement, 7,* 451–472.

Jones, W. H., & Briggs, S. R. (1984). The self–other discrepancy in social shyness. In R. Schwarzer (Ed.), *The self in anxiety, stress, and depression* (pp. 93–108). Amsterdam: North-Holland.

Jussim, L. (1991). Social perception and social reality: A reflection–construction model. *Psychological Review, 98,* 54–73.

Kashy, D. A. (1988). *Intergroup processes: A social relations perspective.* Unpublished master's thesis, University of Connecticut.

Kashy, D. A. (1992). Levels of analysis of social interaction diaries: Separating the effects of person, partner, day, and interaction (Doctoral dissertation, University of Connecticut, 1991). *Dissertation Abstracts International, 53,* 608A.

Kashy, D. A., & Kenny, D. A. (1990a). Do you know whom you were with a week ago Friday? A re-analysis of the Bernard, Killworth, and Sailer studies. *Social Psychology Quarterly, 53,* 55–61.

Kashy, D. A., & Kenny, D. A. (1990b). Analysis of family research designs: A model of interdependence. *Communication Research, 17,* 462–482.

Kelley, H. H., & Stahelski, A. J. (1970). Social interaction basis of cooperators' and competitors' beliefs about others. *Journal of Personality and Social Psychology, 16,* 66–91.

Kelly, G. A. (1955). *The psychology of personal constructs.* New York: Norton.

Kenny, D. A. (1981). Interpersonal perception: A multivariate round robin analysis. In M. B. Brewer & B. F. Collins (Eds.), *Scientific inquiry and the social sciences: A volume in honor of Donald T. Campbell* (pp. 288–309). San Francisco: Jossey-Bass.

Kenny, D. A. (1986). Methods for measuring dyads and groups. In W. D. Crano & M. B. Brewer (Eds.), *Principles and methods of social research* (pp. 301–320). Boston: Allyn & Bacon.

Kenny, D. A. (1988). Interpersonal perception: A social relations analysis. *Journal of Social and Personal Relationships, 5,* 247–261.

Kenny, D. A. (1990). Design issues in dyadic research. In C. Hendrick & M. S. Clark (Eds.), *Review of personality and social psychology: Vol. 11. Research methods in personality and social psychology* (pp. 164–184). Newbury Park, CA: Sage.

Kenny, D. A. (1991). A general model of consensus and accuracy in interpersonal perception. *Psychological Review, 98,* 155–163.

Kenny, D. A. (1992). [Zero acquaintance replication with self-ratings before other ratings.] Unpublished raw data, University of Connecticut.

Kenny, D. A. (1993a). *SOREMO: A FORTRAN program for the analysis of round-robin data structures.* Unpublished manuscript, University of Connecticut.

Kenny, D. A. (1993b). *BLOCKO: A FORTRAN program for the analysis of block data structures.* Unpublished manuscript, University of Connecticut.

Kenny, D. A. (1994). Using the Social Relations Model to understand relationships. In R. Erber & R. Gilmour (Eds.), *Theoretical frameworks for personal relationships* (pp. 111–127). Hillsdale, NJ: Erlbaum.

Kenny, D. A., & Albright, L. (1987). Accuracy in interpersonal perception: A social relations analysis. *Psychological Bulletin, 102,* 390–402.

Kenny, D. A., Albright, L., Malloy, T. E., & Kashy, D. A. (in press). Consensus in interpersonal perception: Acquaintance and the Big Five. *Psychological Bulletin.*

Kenny, D. A., & Bernstein, N. (1982). [Interactions between opposite-sex strangers.] Unpublished raw data, University of Connecticut.

Kenny, D. A., & DePaulo, B. M. (1990). [Applicant-interviewer study.] Unpublished raw data, University of Connecticut.

Kenny, D. A., & DePaulo, B. M. (1993). Do people know how others view them?: An empirical and theoretical account. *Psychological Bulletin, 114,* 145–161.

Kenny, D. A., Horner, C., Kashy, D. A., & Chu, L. (1992). Consensus at zero acquaintance: Replication, behavioral cues, and stability. *Journal of Personality and Social Psychology, 62,* 88–97.

Kenny, D. A., & Judd, C. M. (1986). Consequences of violating the independence assumption in analysis of variance. *Psychological Bulletin, 99,* 422–431.

Kenny, D. A., & Kashy, D. A. (in press). Enhanced coorientation in the perception of friends: A social relations analysis. *Journal of Personality and Social Psychology.*

Kenny, D. A., & La Voie, L. (1982). Reciprocity of interpersonal attraction: A confirmed hypothesis. *Social Psychology Quarterly, 45,* 54–58.

Kenny, D. A., & La Voie, L. (1984). The Social Relations Model. In L. Berkowitz (Ed.), *Advances in experimental social psychology* (Vol. 18, pp. 142–182). Orlando, FL: Academic Press.

Kenny, D. A., & Malloy, T. E. (1988). Partner effects in social interaction. *Journal of Nonverbal Behavior, 12,* 34–57.

Kenny, D. A., & Nasby, W. (1980). Splitting the reciprocity correlation. *Journal of Personality and Social Psychology, 38,* 249–256.

Kenrick, D. T., & Funder, D. C. (1988). Profiting from controversy: Lessons from the person–situation debate. *American Psychologist, 43,* 23–34.

Kenrick, D. T., & Stringfield, D. O. (1980). Personality traits and the eye of the beholder: Crossing some traditional philosophical boundaries in the search for consistency in all of the people. *Psychological Review, 87,* 88–104.

Kinch, J. W. (1963). A formalized theory of the self-concept. *American Journal of Sociology, 68,* 481–486.

Krackhardt, D. (1987). Cognitive social structures. *Social Networks, 9,* 109–134.

Kruglanski, A. W. (1989). The psychology of being "right": The problem of accuracy in social perception and cognition. *Psychological Bulletin, 106,* 395–409.

Laing, R. D., Phillipson, H., & Lee, A. R. (1966). *Interpersonal perception: A theory and a method of research.* New York: Springer.

Latané, B. (1987). [Photo ratings from the CAPS study.] Unpublished raw data, University of North Carolina.

Leary, M. R. (1983). *Understanding social anxiety: Social, personality, and clinical perspectives.* Newbury Park, CA: Sage.

Levesque, M. J. (1990). [Round-robin ratings following mock jury deliberations: Perceptions of intelligence and influence.] Unpublished raw data, University of Connecticut.

Levesque, M. J., & Kenny, D. A. (1993). Accuracy of behavioral predictions at zero acquaintance: A social relations analysis. *Journal of Personality and Social Psychology, 65,* 1178–1187.

Levine, J., & Snyder, H. (1980). [Social perception among five and six year olds.] Unpublished raw data, University of Pittsburgh.

Lewinsohn, P. M., Mischel, W., Chaplin, W., & Barton, R. (1980). Social competence and depression: The role of illusory self-perceptions. *Journal of Abnormal Psychology, 89,* 203–212.

Locksley, A., Borgida, E., Brekke, N., & Hepburn, C. (1980). Sex stereotypes and social judgment. *Journal of Personality and Social Psychology, 39,* 821–831.

Malloy, T. E. (1987a). [A longitudinal study of interpersonal perception.] Unpublished raw data, Rhode Island College.

Malloy, T. E. (1987b). Self-referenced social perception (Doctoral dissertation, University of Connecticut, 1986). *Dissertation Abstracts International, 47,* 4008A.

Malloy, T. E., & Albright, L. (1990). Interpersonal perception in a social context. *Journal of Personality and Social Psychology, 58,* 419–428.

Malloy, T. E., & Janowski, C. L. (1992). Perceptions and metaperceptions of leadership: Components, accuracy, and dispositional correlates. *Personality and Social Psychology Bulletin, 18,* 700–708.

Malloy, T. E., & Kenny, D. A. (1986). The Social Relations Model: An integrative methodology for personality research. *Journal of Personality, 54,* 199–225.

Markus, H. (1977). Self-schemata and processing information about the self. *Journal of Personality and Social Psychology, 35,* 63–78.

Markus, H., & Zajonc, R. B. (1985). The cognitive perspective in social psychology. In G. Lindzey & E. Aronson (Eds.), *The handbook of social psychology* (3rd ed., Vol. 1, pp. 137–230). New York: Random House.

Maslow, A. H. (1954). *Motivation and personality.* New York: Harper.

McArthur, L. Z., & Baron, R. M. (1983). Toward an ecological theory of social perception. *Psychological Review, 90,* 215–238.

McCrae, R. R. (1982). Consensual validation of personality traits: Evidence from self-reports and ratings. *Journal of Personality and Social Psychology, 43,* 293–303.

McCrae, R. R., & Costa, P. T., Jr. (1989). Different points of view: Self-reports and ratings in the assessment of personality. In J. P. Forgas & M. J. Innes (Eds.), *Recent advances in social psychology* (pp. 429–439). Amsterdam: North-Holland.

McGillan, V. (1980). [Sex-role stereotypes and interpersonal behavior.] Unpublished raw data, Clark University.

McHenry, R. (1971). New methods of assessing accuracy in person perception. *Journal of the Theory of Social Behaviour, 1,* 109–119.

McLeod, J., & Chaffee, S. H. (1973). Interpersonal approaches to communication research. *American Behavioral Scientist, 16,* 467–500.

Mead, G. H. (1925). The genesis of the self and social control. *International Journal of Ethics, 35,* 251–273.

Mead, G. H. (1934). *Mind, self, and society.* Chicago: University of Chicago Press.

Merton, R. K. (1957). *Social theory and social structure.* Glencoe, IL: Free Press.

Montgomery, B. (1984). Individual differences and relational interdependences in social interaction. *Human Communication Research, 11,* 33–60.

Moskowitz, D. S., & Schwarz, J. C. (1982). Validity comparison of behavior counts and ratings by knowledgeable informants. *Journal of Personality and Social Psychology, 42,* 518–528.

Newcomb, T. M. (1961). *The acquaintance process.* New York: Holt, Rinehart & Winston.

Newcomb, T. M. (1979). Reciprocity of interpersonal attraction: A nonconfirmation of a plausible hypothesis. *Social Psychology Quarterly, 42,* 299–306.

Nisbett, R. E., & Ross, L. (1980). *Human inference: Strategies and shortcomings of social judgment.* Englewood Cliffs, NJ: Prentice-Hall.

Nisbett, R. E., & Wilson, T. D. (1977). Telling more than we can know: Verbal reports on mental processes. *Psychological Review, 84,* 231–259.

Norman, W. T. (1963). Toward an adequate taxonomy of personality attributes: Replicated factor structure in peer nomination personality ratings. *Journal of Abnormal and Social Psychology, 66,* 574–583.

Norman, W. T., & Goldberg, L. R. (1966). Raters, ratees, and randomness in personality structure. *Journal of Personality and Social Psychology, 4,* 681–691.

Nunnally, J. (1967). *Psychometric theory.* New York: McGraw-Hill.

Oliver, P. V. (1989). Effects of need for social approval on first interaction among members of the opposite sex (Doctoral dissertation, University of Connecticut, 1988). *Dissertation Abstracts International, 50,* 1155A.

Park, B. (1986). A method for studying the development of impressions of real people. *Journal of Personality and Social Psychology, 51,* 907–917.

Park, B., DeKay, M. L., & Kraus, S. (1994). Aggregating social behavior into person models: Perceiver-induced consistency. *Journal of Personality and Social Psychology, 66,* 437–459.

Park, B., & Flink, C. (1989). A social relations analysis of agreement in liking judgments. *Journal of Personality and Social Psychology, 56,* 506–518.

Park, B., & Judd, C. M. (1989). Agreement on initial impressions: Differences due to perceivers, trait dimensions, and target behaviors. *Journal of Personality and Social Psychology, 56,* 493–505.

Paulhus, D. L., & Bruce, M. N. (1992). The effect of acquaintanceship on the validity of personality impressions: A longitudinal study. *Journal of Personality and Social Psychology, 63,* 816–824.

Paunonen, S. V. (1989). Consensus in personality judgments: Moderating effects of target–rater acquaintanceship and behavior observability. *Journal of Personality and Social Psychology, 56,* 823–833.

Paunonen, S. V., & Jackson, D. N. (1985). Idiographic measurement strategies for personality and prediction: Some unredeemed promissory notes. *Psychological Review, 92,* 486–511.

Pennington, N., & Hastie, R. (1991). A cognitive theory of juror decision making: The story model. *Cardozo Law Review, 13,* 5001–5039.

Pozo, C., Carver, C. S., Wellens, A. R., & Scheier, M. F. (1991). Social anxiety and social perception: Construing others' reactions to self. *Personality and Social Psychology Bulletin, 17,* 355–362.

Read, S. J., & Miller, L. C. (1993). Rapist or "regular guy": Explanatory coherence in the construction of mental models of others. *Personality and Social Psychology Bulletin, 19,* 526–540.

Reeder, G. D., & Brewer, M. B. (1979). A schematic model of dispositional attribution in interpersonal perception. *Psychological Review, 86,* 61–79.

Reno, R. R., & Kenny, D. A. (1992). Effects of self-consciousness and social anxiety on self-disclosure among unacquainted individuals: An application of the Social Relations Model. *Journal of Personality, 60,* 79–94.

Richards, J. M., Jr., & Cline, V. B. (1963). Accuracy components in person perception scores and the scoring system as an artifact in investigations of the generality of judging ability. *Psychological Reports, 12,* 363–373.

Romney, A. K., Weller, S. C., & Batchelder, W. H. (1986). Culture as consensus: A theory of culture and informant accuracy. *American Anthropologist, 88,* 313–338.

Rosenberg, S. (1986). Self-concept for middle childhood through adolescence. In J. Suls & A. G. Greenwald (Eds.), *Psychological perspectives on the self* (Vol. 3, pp. 107–136). Hillsdale, NJ: Erlbaum.

Rosengren, W. R. (1961). The self in the emotionally disturbed. *American Journal of Sociology, 66,* 454–462.

Rosenthal, R., Hall, J. A., DiMatteo, M. R., Rogers, P. L., & Archer, D. (1979). *Sensitivity to nonverbal communication: The PONS test.* Baltimore: Johns Hopkins University Press.

Rosenthal, R. (1966). *Experimenter effects in behavioral research.* New York: Appleton-Century-Crofts.

Ross, H. S., & Lollis, S. P. (1989). A social relations analysis of toddler peer relationships. *Child Development, 60,* 1082–1091.

Ross, L., Greene, D., & House, P. (1977). The false consensus effect: An egocentric bias in social perception and attribution processes. *Journal of Experimental Social Psychology, 13,* 279–301.

Ross, L., & Nisbett, R. E. (1991). *The person and the situation: Perspectives of social psychology.* New York: McGraw-Hill.

Rothbart, M., & Singer, B. (1988). [Peer-ratings in an ingroup–outgroup study.] Unpublished raw data, University of Oregon.

Rozelle, R. M., & Baxter, J. C. (1981). Influence of role pressures on the perceiver: Judgments of videotaped interviews varying judge accountability and responsibility. *Journal of Applied Psychology, 66,* 437–441.

Scheff, T. J. (1967). Toward a sociological model of consensus. *American Sociological Review, 32,* 32–46.

Schill, T., & Thomsen, D. (1987). Anger, hostility, and the Barron ego strength scale. *Psychological Reports, 60,* 1113–1114.

Schlenker, B. R. (1980). *Impression management.* Monterey, CA: Brooks/Cole.

Schlenker, B. R. (1985). *The self and social life.* New York: McGraw-Hill.

Schlenker, B. R., & Leary, M. R. (1982). Social anxiety and self-presentation: A conceptualization and model. *Psychological Bulletin, 92,* 641–669.

Schneider, D. J., Hastorf, A. H., & Ellsworth, P. C. (1979). *Person perception* (2nd ed.). Reading, MA: Addison-Wesley.

Shechtman, Z. (1994). *Agreement between lay participants and professional assessors: A study of a group assessment procedure for teacher-candidate selection.* Unpublished manuscript, Haifa University, Haifa, Israel.

Shechtman, Z., & Kenny, D. A. (in press). Meta-perception accuracy: An Israeli study. *Journal of Basic and Applied Social Psychology.*

Shrauger, J. S., & Schoeneman, T. J. (1979). Symbolic interactionist view of self-concept: Through the looking glass darkly. *Psychological Bulletin, 86,* 549–573.

Smith, H. C. (1966). *Sensitivity to people.* New York: McGraw-Hill.

Snodgrass, S. E. (1985). Women's intuition: The effect of subordinate role on interpersonal sensitivity. *Journal of Personality and Social Psychology, 49,* 146–155.

Snodgrass, S. E. (1992). Further effects of role versus gender on interpersonal sensitivity. *Journal of Personality and Social Psychology, 62,* 154–158.

Snyder, M. (1974). Self-monitoring of expressive behavior. *Journal of Personality and Social Psychology, 30,* 526–537.

Snyder, M. (1979). Self-monitoring processes. In L. Berkowitz (Ed.), *Advances in experimental social psychology* (Vol. 12, pp. 85–128). New York: Academic Press.

Snyder, M., & Swann, W. B., Jr. (1978). Behavioral confirmation in social interaction: From social perception to social reality. *Journal of Experimental Social Psychology, 14,* 148–162.

Stanley, J. C. (1961). Analysis of unreplicated three-way classifications, with applications to rater bias and trait independence. *Psychometrika, 26,* 205–219.

Steiner, I. (1955). Interpersonal behavior as influenced by accuracy of social perception. *Psychological Review, 62,* 268–274.

Surra, C. A., & Ridley, C. A. (1991). Multiple perspectives on interaction: Participants, peers, and observers. In B. M. Montgomery & S. Duck (Eds.),
Studying interpersonal interaction (pp. 35–55). New York: Guilford Press.

Swann, W. B., Jr. (1984). Quest for accuracy in person perception: A matter of
pragmatics. *Psychological Review, 91,* 457–477.

Swann, W. B., Jr. (1990). To be adored or to be known? The interplay of self-
enhancement and self-verification. In E. T. Higgins & R. M. Sorrentino (Eds.),
Handbook of motivation and cognition: Foundations of social behavior (Vol.
2, pp. 408–448). New York: Guilford Press.

Swann, W. B., Jr., & Ely, R. J. (1984). A battle of wills: Self-verification versus
behavioral confirmation. *Journal of Personality and Social Psychology, 46,*
1287–1302.

Swann, W. B., Jr., & Hill, C. A. (1982). When our identities are mistaken:
Reaffirming self-conceptions through social interaction. *Journal of Personality and Social Psychology, 43,* 59–66.

Swann, W. B., Jr., & Predmore, S. C. (1985). Intimates as agents of social support: Sources of consolation or despair? *Journal of Personality and Social Psychology, 49,* 1609–1617.

Swann, W. B., Jr., Stein-Seroussi, A., & McNulty, S. E. (1992). Outcasts in a
white-lie society: The enigmatic worlds of people with negative self-
conceptions. *Journal of Personality and Social Psychology, 62,* 618–624.

Tagiuri, R. (1969). Person perception. In G. Lindzey & E. Aronson (Eds.), *Handbook of social psychology* (2nd ed., Vol. 3, pp. 395–449). Reading, MA:
Addison-Wesley.

Tagiuri, R., Bruner, J. S., & Blake, R. R. (1958). On the relation between feelings and perception of feelings among members of small groups. In E. E. Mac-
coby, T. M. Newcomb, & E. L. Hartley (Eds.), *Readings in social psychology*
(3rd ed., pp. 110–116). New York: Holt, Rinehart & Winston.

Tannen, D. (1990). *You just don't understand: Women and men in conversation.*
New York: Morrow.

Taylor, S. E., & Brown, J. D. (1988). Illusion and well-being: A social psychological perspective on mental health. *Psychological Bulletin, 103,* 193–210.

Tedeschi, J. T. (1981). *Impression management theory and social psychological
research.* New York: Academic Press.

Teglasi, H., & Hoffman, M. A. (1982). Causal attributions of shy subjects. *Journal
of Research in Personality, 16,* 376–385.

Tesser, A., & Rosen, S. (1975). The reluctance to transmit bad news. In L. Berkowitz (Ed.), *Advances in experimental social psychology* (Vol. 8, pp.
194–232). Orlando, FL: Academic Press.

Touhey, J. C. (1972). Role perception and the relative influence of the perceiver
and the perceived. *Journal of Social Psychology, 87,* 213–217.

Trope, Y., & Higgins, E. T. (1993). The what, when, and how of dispositional inference: New answers and new questions. *Personality and Social Psychology Bulletin, 19,* 493–500.

Warner, R., Kenny, D. A., & Stoto, M. (1979). A new round robin analysis of variance for social interaction data. *Journal of Personality and Social Psychology, 37,* 1742–1757.

Whitley, B. E., Schofield, J. W., & Snyder, H. N. (1984). Peer preferences in a desegregated school: A round robin analysis. *Journal of Personality and Social Psychology, 46,* 799–810.

Wiggins, J. S. (1973). *Personality and prediction: Principles of personality assessment.* Reading, MA: Addison-Wesley.

Wilson, T. D., Hull, J. G., & Johnson, J. (1981). Awareness and self-perception: Verbal reports on internal states. *Journal of Personality and Social Psychology, 40,* 53–71.

Winter, L., & Uleman, J. S. (1984). When are social judgments made? Evidence for the spontaneousness of trait inferences. *Journal of Personality and Social Psychology, 17,* 237–252.

Woodruffe, C. (1984). The consistency of presented personality: Additional evidence from aggregation. *Journal of Personality, 52,* 307–317.

Wright, T. L., Ingraham, L. J., & Blackmer, D. R. (1985). Simultaneous study of individual differences and relationship effects in attraction. *Journal of Personality and Social Psychology, 47,* 1059–1062.

Wyer, R. S., Jr., Henninger, M., & Wolfson, M. (1975). Informational determinants of females' self-attributions and observers' judgments of them in an achievement situation. *Journal of Personality and Social Psychology, 32,* 556–570.

Yingling, J. (1989). *Interpersonal communication competence: Contributions of individual tendency and relational context.* Unpublished manuscript, University of Northern Colorado.

Yzerbyt, V. (1988). [Ingroup–outgroup perceptions.] Unpublished data analyses, Louvain University, Louvain, Belgium.

Zaccaro, S., Foti, R. J., & Kenny, D. A. (1991). Self-monitoring and trait-based variance in leadership: An investigation of leader flexibility across multiple group situations. *Journal of Applied Psychology, 76,* 308–315.

Zajonc, R. B. (1980). Feeling and thinking: Preferences need no inferences. *American Psychologist, 35,* 151–175.

Zebrowitz, L. A. (1990). *Social perception.* Pacific Grove, CA: Brooks/Cole.

Zuckerman, Marvin, Kuhlman, D. M., Joireman, J., Teta, P., & Kraft, M. (1993). A comparison of three structural models for personality: The Big Three, the Big Five, and the Alternative Five. *Journal of Personality and Social Psychology, 65,* 757–768.

Zuckerman, Miron, Koestner, R., & Alton, A. O. (1984). Learning to detect deception. *Journal of Personality and Social Psychology, 46,* 519–528.

INDEX

CPSIA information can be obtained
at www.ICGtesting.com
Printed in the USA
LVOW12*1424071216

516242LV00006B/74/P

9 780898 621143